5.18.16
#17.99

AS

Withdrawn

Kokoro Yoga

8 Weeks to SEALFIT:
A Navy SEAL's Guide to Unconventional Training for Physical and
Mental Toughness

Unbeatable Mind:
Forge Resiliency and Mental Toughness to Succeed at an Elite Level

The Way of the SEAL:
Think Like an Elite Warrior to Lead and Succeed (with Allyson E. Machate)

MAXIMIZE YOUR HUMAN POTENTIAL AND DEVELOP THE SPIRIT OF A WARRIOR

kokoro

yoga

MARK DIVINE
CDR, U.S. Navy SEAL

and CATHERINE DIVINE

Foreword by Gary Kraftsow

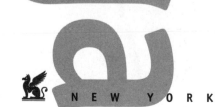 ST. MARTIN'S GRIFFIN 🦅 NEW YORK

The information in this book is not intended to replace the advice of the reader's own physician or other medical professional. You should consult a medical professional in matters relating to health, especially if you have existing medical conditions, and before starting any new fitness regimen. The author and the publisher do not accept responsibility for any adverse effects individuals may claim to experience, whether directly or indirectly, from the information contained in this book.

KOKORO YOGA. Copyright © 2016 by Mark Divine and Catherine Divine. Foreword © 2016 by Gary Kraftsow. All rights reserved. Printed in the United States of America. For information, address St. Martin's Press, 175 Fifth Avenue, New York, N.Y. 10010.

Designed by Richard Oriolo

Library of Congress Cataloging-in-Publication Data

Names: Divine, Mark. author. | Divine, Catherine, author.
Title: Kokoro yoga : maximize your human potential and develop the spirit of
   a warrior / by CDR Mark Divine, US Navy SEAL, and Catherine Divine;
   foreword by Gary Kraftsow.
Description: New York, NY : St. Martin's Griffin, 2016.
Identifiers: LCCN 2015045659| ISBN 9781250067210 (paperback) | ISBN
   9781466875227 (e-book)
Subjects: LCSH: Yoga. | Mental health. | Mind and body. | BISAC: HEALTH &
   FITNESS / Yoga. | SELF-HELP / Motivational & Inspirational.
Classification: LCC B132.Y6 D575 2016 | DDC 613.7/046—dc23
LC record available at http://lccn.loc.gov/2015045659

Our books may be purchased in bulk for promotional, educational, or business use. Please contact your local bookseller or the Macmillan Corporate and Premium Sales Department at 1-800-221-7945, extension 5442, or by e-mail at MacmillanSpecialMarkets@macmillan.com.

First Edition: April 2016

10 9 8 7 6 5 4 3 2

CONTENTS

Yoga is growing in popularity worldwide at an unprecedented rate. The great majority of enthusiasts and practitioners, however, primarily see yoga as a system of exercise oriented toward development of the physical body through the performance of postures known as asana.

To a lesser extent, but increasing steadily, is the emergence of the field of "yoga therapy" as a system of self-care. Perhaps one of the most significant roles of yoga therapy in the context of modern health care is helping with the paradigm shift from illness-based and health practitioner–based care to wellness-based and self-based care.

The scope of yoga therapy extends from:

- A form of adapted movement therapy to manage structural conditions to

- A method of sympathetic/parasympathetic regulation via specialized breathing practices to help manage common symptoms of chronic illness such as stress, sleeplessness, fatigue, and pain management to

- A system of mental health care via an integrated use of breathing practices, self-inquiry, and meditation to help balance emotions, clarify thoughts, and support behavioral change.

Modern scientific and medical research is demonstrating the incredible health benefits of these practices for anatomy, physiology, and the brain. Beyond these more physical benefits, the deeper work of yoga helps us surface our unconscious patterns, gain control over our desires, feelings, thoughts, and behavior. Through these practices we can deepen our self-understanding and gain mastery over our bodies and minds. With that as a foundation, we can access the higher states of awareness that lead to deep wisdom and compassion, and enable us to tap into and actualize our highest potential.

Mark Divine speaks from this deeper and more integrated understanding of yoga in

Kokoro Yoga. While yoga therapy can function as a kind of life raft, helping those lost in the ocean of suffering, Kokoro Yoga is a kind of a launchpad for those who want to blast off into the unexplored regions of their own potential.

Sharing his own personal journey from would-be Wall Street professional, to martial artist, to Navy SEAL, to creator of SEALFIT, Mark clearly illustrates the power of the integrated approach to self-development passed on by the ancients.

As a starting point, Mark shares with us his self-reflections that "his career path was incongruent with his ideals." This insight initiated his journey of self-discovery and self-development. From martial arts training to Navy SEAL training, he continues to listen to his inner voice. "Though trained to kill," he shares, his heart led him to "discover the path of the peaceful warrior."

Mark lays out the foundation of this path throughout his book, linking his own insight and understanding to ancient yogic teachings drawn from key texts such as the *Bhagavad Gita,* the Yoga Sutras of *Patanjali,* and the *Taittiriya Upanishad.* He explains the importance and necessity of building an ethical foundation as the root of self-development. He systematically walks us through the component parts of integrated self-development, including training the body, the breath, and the mind. He emphasizes key characteristics of the successful warrior, including the ability to stay "calm, energized, in control of one's emotions, focused, ready for the mission, and able to manage the stress" that arises in any situation.

Mark reflects on his own experience as he gets older, and the importance of continually rebalancing his training to avoid injuries and burnout. Through his ongoing reflective self-awareness as he trains, he realizes what the ancients said: Our practice must change and evolve to reflect our own stage in life.

Early in the book, Mark speaks of a saying among the SEALs, "Take care of your gear, and it will take care of you." Similarly, the ancient yogis used to say, "Take care of dharma, and dharma will take care of you." As I read through Mark's book, it became clear that he has truly realized this ideal. Mark's personal journey on the path of Kokoro Yoga, working multidimensionally to optimize his potential at every level—physical, mental, emotional, intuitive, and spiritual—led to his discovery of his own *svadharma* and self-definition as a "world-centric warrior and servant of humanity." A true yogi, Mark has realized through his own efforts that the purpose of human development leading to self-mastery is altruistic; that we then are able to serve others better!

This book explains clearly what self-development means at each level. It offers clear training instructions and tactics that will guide those committed to an ongoing path of self-development and personal growth. More than anything else, this book is a manual for self-empowerment, sharing in contemporary language an ancient path that enables each individual to actualize his or her potential and live life with meaning and purpose.

—Gary Kraftsow
Author of *Yoga for Wellness* and *Yoga for Transformation*
December 2015
Oakland, California

Kokoro Yoga

CHAPTER 1

AN M4 AND A YOGA MAT

My path to a complete warrior art

In the beginner's mind there are many possibilities, but in the expert's there are very few.
— SHUNRYU SUZUKI

INTO THE BREACH

IN 1991 I WAS A NAVY OFFICER, RECENTLY GRADUATED FROM SEAL TRAINING (BUD/S) AS THE HONOR MAN IN MY CLASS, EARNING THE COVETED NAVY SEAL TRIDENT. SOON I WAS ASSIGNED TO SEAL TEAM 3, TASKED TO GO TO IRAQ TO FIGHT IN OPERATION DESERT STORM. FORTUNATELY FOR MANY, THAT WAR ENDED BEFORE WE DEPLOYED, and at SEAL Team 3 I would complete 6 more years of active duty in a relatively peaceful period of our history. Although I would visit the Middle East a number of times from 1991 to 1997, I wouldn't get the call to go to another turbulent Iraq until 2004, when I was serving as a reserve officer.

Like most in the reserves during that time, it wasn't a surprise for me to get mobilized for duty during what was being called the war on terror. I knew it was coming but was not sure when.

At 41, my days as a gun-slinging operator were behind me. It didn't make sense for me to go back to a shooting SEAL task unit. So it was cool that my mission would be to lead a fairly complicated study for the U.S. Navy, involving the integration of the U.S. Marine Corps (USMC) into the special ops community (also known as SOCOM). I was to shadow a detachment of 100 handpicked U.S. Marines, intelligence and recon guys called SOCOM Detachment 1 who were to conduct a proof-of-concept deployment under the watchful eyes of SEAL Team 1.

It was a big deal. Twenty years earlier, the Marines had declined to be a part of the joint program to form the Special Operations Command, which included the Navy's SEAL teams, the Army's special forces and a Ranger battalion, and the Air Force's special ops teams such as Pararescue. But after 9/11, as the Marine Corps watched particularly hot missions—and the money to support them—flow to SOCOM, they started to rethink their position. The secretary of defense, Donald Rumsfeld, put the brakes on an effort to fast-track the process. He didn't want to mess around with the 20 years of intricate and complicated coordination work that had already happened between the initial units of SOCOM. A thorough study and evaluation was deemed important to make sure that they didn't screw up what had taken years to get to work well. Though the USMC was ready to throw the 100-man team into combat, validation was a good idea before sending a newly formed concept team from a conventional-minded military service into the murky SOF (Special Operations Forces) world. And as you might imagine, there were a lot of charged convictions and emotions when it came to who was taking orders from whom between the SEALs and Marines. The call I got for the job was from Commander Mike Lumpkin, who was then the Naval Special Warfare Group 1 operations officer and had just rolled out of the position as deputy commander of Special Operations Forces, overseeing the 2,000 special operators in Baghdad. (In 2013, Mike Lumpkin became the assistant secretary of defense for SOLIC.)

Prior to deployment to the combat zone with SEAL Team 1, I would lead the organization of the predeployment training certification for SEAL Team 1 with the 100 U.S. Marines from

SOCOM Det 1 in tow. This was a good project for me. For one thing, I was intrigued with the underlying matrix of leadership that would need to be worked out between the SEALs and the Marines. Since my years on SEAL Team 3, I had expanded my views and beliefs regarding the definition of a "warrior," leaving behind most parochial and tribal viewpoints on who is the best branch of the military, or who is the best special operator. Even though I was a SEAL, through and through, I would be able to offer an impartial viewpoint in conducting the exercise and ensuing study. My job was made easy by the fact that the Marines were great guys and solid operators

The certification exercise was a big success, and the time finally came for me to deploy to Baghdad to continue part two of my job, the study of the Marine team in SOF combat. Things happened fast. I paid a visit to the supply depot in Coronado, California, to get my weapon and gear, said good-bye to my family, and before I knew it I was on a flight to Bahrain—with a bunch of polished new gear and an M4 rifle that I hadn't had time to take to the range. As an active-duty SEAL, shooting "my" weapon seemed to be a constant. I got real intimate with my primary and secondary weapons. But in the reserves we did not get issued our own weapons, so I literally had to check one out of the armory before I left. Any military member will understand how important it is to sight in your weapon and get comfortable with its idiosyncrasies. In addition, the life of the active-duty SEAL involves around-the-clock training and sharpening skills as an individual and as part of a team. It is a day-in, day-out, year-round affair. As an officer in the SEAL reserves, however, we didn't get to shoot nearly as much, nor did we get issued our own weapon to sleep with.

That was a big concern of mine, along with the web gear I was to use. I had brand-new web gear that wasn't broken in and customized to fit my frame. I needed to "run and gun" with the gear to ensure I would know where the ammo pouches would be in a pinch, and to make sure they wouldn't fly off in a firefight. On active duty, I got really comfortable with my equipment and knew I could rely on it. We had a saying: "Take care of your gear, and it will take care of you!" But here I was, about to deploy into a war zone, and I was looking at a bunch of plastic bags encasing brand-new, untouched equipment and a weapon I hadn't even shot yet. My pucker factor—military jargon for adrenalin—was rising.

Ratcheting up the stress was the news coming out of Iraq. On March 31, 2004, a friend of mine, Stephen "Scott" Helvenston, was one of four Blackwater military contractors that were in a convoy ambushed by insurgents in Fallujah. Scott and the others were killed in a horrifying manner, made worse for me by the fact that I saw him the day before he deployed weeks earlier. This was to be his last deployment with Blackwater. The graphic imagery startled me, knowing that I would soon be stepping into that same area where I could easily be the next target.

To make matters even worse, in mid-May, days before my deployment, a militant group posted a video of the decapitation of Nick Berg, an American radio-tower repairman from Pennsylvania. The video, which I immediately regretted watching, made me sick to my stomach. The stark reminder that we were fighting an enemy who seemed nuts, believing they were in the right to perform such deranged and hideous acts, steeled me as I stepped onto the C-130.

On my way to Baghdad, I stopped in Bahrain for a couple of days while awaiting final transport to the war zone. There I met up with a civilian analyst, from the Center for Naval Analysis, assigned to write the USMC side of the same report I was working on. He was to go to the Green Zone (the so-called secure area in Baghdad that the American military worked) with me. We discussed the project and our approaches as we waited for our ride.

The C-130 was scheduled to depart at 0500 hours. As I waited for the analyst to share a ride to the airfield, he approached me and said, "Mark, I won't be going. I have a bad feeling about this." Great, I thought, . . . Wonder if he knows something I don't!

Well, I was going anyhow. I couldn't lose face with my teammates and I was a tough SEAL officer, right? Climbing aboard the turboprop transport workhorse, the C-130, which the U.S. military uses to transport troops and equipment, I was never more nervous in my life. Keenly aware that anything could happen I felt on high alert. As the windowless C-130 roared into the air, I considered how things were stacking up. My civilian counterpart may have been spooked by another story in the press of how an Australian soldier had caught a bullet through his ass while on an aircraft leaving Baghdad. It was just someone shooting from the ground. A bullet had ripped through the fuselage and killed him. The ominous signs were getting the best of me.

Sitting across from me was a one-star Marine general working feverishly on a presentation with an aide. It was a 2-hour flight. After we lifted off, I couldn't bear sitting so I looked around the plane and spotted an open space by some cargo netting in the ramp area. My thoughts were set to full speed and I needed to do something to calm down. Remembering how calm I felt after my yoga sessions back home, I went to the open space near a stack of pallets and started doing a deep-breathing exercise and a few forward folds and backbends. This led to a full-blown yoga session in the middle of the bumpy ride in the C-130. (Later in my reserve career, I made it a point to practice yoga on military transports whenever I could. Often I had other members of my SEAL team or other military passengers join me, but I am pretty sure this was a first in military history!) The one-star Marine general must have been thinking: That SEAL officer is obviously green to combat and scared shitless. I didn't care. The yoga began to calm my mind and helped me regain control of my emotions. I felt much better as we turned our nose toward the Iraqi desert.

By the time we landed in Baghdad, I wasn't in a perfect Zen state by any means—we were in a combat zone after all—but I was far more calm, present, and centered, and ready for what came next.

That was a good thing. I hadn't been on the ground more than 15 minutes when I heard someone shout, "Incoming!," followed by the unmistakable whistle of a mortar flying toward us. I had only heard mortars while in training, not combat, and in training they are whistling away from you. Trust me when I say it sounds very different when it is coming full bore at you! It exploded about a quarter mile away. Okay, I said to myself. Welcome to combat.

Later, a couple of SEAL team guys drove up to retrieve me—loaded for bear for the 45-minute ride through bad-guy land—they gave me a sign to lock and load my M4 (I didn't have the guts to tell them I hadn't even sighted it in yet) and off we went to the SEAL compound at one of Saddam Hussein's former palace grounds.

That yoga session on the C-130 was my first official session of what I called Warrior Yoga (I later changed the name to Kokoro Yoga to avoid a trademark infringement). I realized in that moment that yoga presented a powerful toolkit for my own warrior development.

SEIDO: THE BEGINNING OF MY JOURNEY

So there I was, breathing slowly and deeply into a Sun Salutation in the cargo area of a C-130 on my way to a combat zone. I was too focused on the moment to ask the obvious question: How did I get here?

As random and seemingly out of place my initial session of Kokoro Yoga might sound, it was a significant point of arrival in a long and steady search I had been conducting both during my active-duty time with the SEALs and after.

The search was in some ways a circular one, trying to reconnect with the kind of integrated warrior training that had initially infused me with the awareness and courage to let go of a big-money CPA career I had taking shape on Wall Street for the rigorous challenge of becoming and being a Navy SEAL. It started with what had been a growing sense of inner doubt about what I was setting out to do with my life, a voice I largely ignored as I began to climb the corporate ladder. I was in it for the money, in other words. The prospects for my success were bright. One of the chief rewards came from my family who appreciated that I was conforming to an ideal they had for me. Although I wasn't acknowledging it at the time, my career was incongruent with my ideal. There was a growing weight on my shoulders as my future in high finance stretched out before me. I was walking home one night from work when my train of thought was disrupted by a series of shouts coming from a second-floor window of a seven-story building on West 23rd Street. Intrigued, I walked up a flight of stairs and into what would become a truly disruptive force in my life: the Seido Karate dojo run by Grandmaster Tadashi Nakamura.

Nakamura had formerly been deployed to the United States from Japan to lead a style of karate known for tournament fighting, Kyokushinkai. Nakamura had become disenchanted with the lack of dimension in the training and left despite intense pressure from Japan. Nakamura went about creating Seido Karate with the intent of focusing on human development rather than sheer fighting prowess. The word *seido* is Japanese for "sincere way." This was my first exposure to the martial arts, and I soon found that Seido was a practice that truly integrated body, mind, and spirit training. Unlike other martial arts I would become acquainted with over the years, Seido was unique in that it didn't just talk about the mental and spiritual aspects—it was actually part of the training. Meditation and spiritual talks and discussions on mental development were part of the routine, along with the fighting practice. It was through this work that I was able to connect with the sincere voice within my being and understand that I was meant for something different than taking a place in the family business, as was expected.

Seido not only unlatched access to an inner wisdom that led me to join the Navy and become a SEAL, it also prepared me in a foundational way for what is considered the most arduous and demanding military training program in the world.

The five guiding principles of Seido Karate training are as follows:

1. **ETHICAL FOUNDATION.** The ethical foundation of Seido is based upon what's called "bushido," also known as the Way of the Warrior, a series of moral standards embraced by samurai warriors, like honor, frugality, and loyalty. As you read the next chapter in this book, you'll note that the first two levels of yoga, or limbs, are also staked in an ethical foundation.

2. **INTEGRATED DEVELOPMENT.** As mentioned, Seido didn't just pay lip service to the concept of integrating mental and spiritual training into the daily practice,

Nakamura emphasized this fusion: "My purpose in founding Seido Karate was to show what I feel is the true essence, the kernel of true karate: the training of body, mind, and spirit together in order to realize the fullness of human potential."

3. **SPIRITUAL AWARENESS.** Zen meditation is core to the Seido practice. As esoteric as this may sound, the meditation and spiritual lectures helped me develop the awareness and humility to thrive through the ego-busting stress of BUD/S and Hell Week.

4. **CRUCIBLE TRAINING.** Frequent tests and challenges are part of the Seido program and work to help push students to new levels of performance and to comprehend the magnitude of the potential lying within. For example, an annual crucible session at the dojo might include thousands of kicks and punches. Another common crucible session was conducted over the course of days at a monastery, where we would fill our days endlessly cycling back and forth from meditation to karate work.

5. **FORGING MENTAL TOUGHNESS.** In Seido, we were worked hard and steadily toward developing resiliency and a mentally tough attitude where we never backed down. As Nakamura explained: "Seido seeks to develop in each student a 'non-quitting' spirit. No matter what the obstacle or difficulty—emotional, physical, financial— we want students to feel that, though there may be setbacks, they will never be overcome by any of these problems."

The unified training of Seido proved to be invaluable the day I stepped onto the path to become a Navy SEAL. Because of the relentless difficulty of BUD/S, of having to go 100 mph for the better part of a year, from Hell Week to drownproofing to SEAL Qualification Training, I survived the staggeringly high failure rate. Actually it was because of the integrated warrior training, which I took so seriously, that I did more than just survive. I was able to thrive, finishing as honor man, # 1 graduate, of my class.

SEARCH FOR A COMPLETE WARRIOR ART

In joining the Navy SEALs, I was leaving Wall Street behind—a good thing for me. A sacrifice, however, was leaving behind my training at the Seido World Headquarters on West 23rd Street in Manhattan. In departing for the SEALs, I took with me a desire to find another practice that had a similar comprehensive approach to human development that Seido did. Being on a SEAL team was all that I had imagined, of course. But as an operator you get very focused, for obvious reasons, on shooting, fighting, and mission success. You won't find time dedicated to a spiritual practice on the schedule. So my search for something similar to Seido put me on a quest.

SCARS (Special Combat Aggressive Reactionary System) was my first stop. SCARS was developed by a Vietnam vet named Jerry Peterson from a lethal hand-to-hand combat system called Kung Fu San Soo. Peterson had stripped away all of the cultural elements into what you might call a clear science of how to offensively fight to win. The training was brutal—a 30-day, 10-hour-day program to become certified to teach SCARS. I loved the techniques and the training was fun, but whereas Seido was about developing moral character and spirit, SCARS was about fighting and surviving. In fact, SCARS training came with a warning: Do not use unless someone must die. In the end, I had more than 1,000 hours of training in SCARS when I left the active-duty SEAL teams. In a story that illuminates why I was motivated to continue my search for another Seido-like program, my wife, Sandy, had become a therapist for the Navy. One assignment sent her to a U.S. Navy vessel in Australia that would soon be returning home. Her job was to help the sailors prepare for the jarring realities of returning to civilian life after months at sea. At a dinner in the officers' cabin, the commander of the ship was asking about Sandy's background, and it came up that she was married to someone also in the Navy.

"Who are you married to?" she was asked.

"Lieutenant Commander Mark Divine," Sandy answered.

One of the junior officers went off: "Mark Divine! Mark Divine. I know him . . . he's a SEAL and SCARS master. He could kill us all with his pinky finger!"

After I finished laughing when Sandy told me this story, I began to think about it. As much as I didn't want to be known as some sort of CPA to be feared in a corporate audit, I also didn't find it appealing to be known as a master of the science of killing. I knew that humble warriors are the last to pick up a weapon. I was becoming a more peaceful warrior, even as a SEAL officer.

In transitioning from active duty to the SEAL reserve force, I started training in a Goju-Ryu karate dojo, which had similar roots to Seido. I earned my black belt quickly, in part because I already knew most of the physical moves. But there was no meditation or spiritual training, and when I was recalled in 1999 back to active duty for a stint in Egypt and the Middle East, I never returned to Goju-Ryu.

After the 1-year tour of duty, Sandy and I adopted our son, Devon, and moved to North County, San Diego, about a 40-minute drive up the coast from the SEAL base in Coronado. My search continued. I began to study with Sensei Shane Phelps, a ninjutsu master. Sensei Phelps was trying to get his ninjutsu studio, Temple of the Full Autumn Moon, off the ground when I started training with him. I helped him write a business plan, in fact. He had one of the most sensational backgrounds you're ever going to find. He fought in the Vietnam War and then went on to serve 7 years as a Navy SEAL. He worked for the United Nations as a peacekeeper in places like Syria and Lebanon, and also as an antiterrorism agent of the CIA. He got his BA at Stanford went on to earn a masters degree in comparative religion at Harvard and a Master of Divinity at Yale. Before his Western schooling in the Ivy League, however, he spent 2 years studying Tai Chi and meditating at a Buddhist monastery in China. Shane has long been an awesome example of what I call the 20x factor.

To this day I love the art of ninjutsu. It is an incredible combination of some 40 different types of martial arts, with a variety of weapons and both internally (oriented toward the psychological and spiritual) and externally oriented arts (the more physical-leaning of the martial arts). In the negative column, I found the training frustratingly slow-going and fragmented. I was working toward my black belt when Shane's school suddenly ran out of money and closed its doors. He began working with only private clients, and so my search continued for the complete warrior workout.

It was during this phase of my journey when I discovered yoga.

THE WAY OF THE PEACEFUL WARRIOR

Yoga in the West is viewed through a variety of lenses . . . for most it is a form of exercise. Pilates, Power Yoga, Core Yoga, and Hot Yoga are good examples of this movement. Others may consider it a mystical practice bound to Hinduism, or as a place to train Cirque du Soleil athletes. Since the late 1990s there has been a boom of yoga studios around the country giving rise to millions walking to and from group classes with mats jutting out of their backpacks in a quest to stretch, bend, sweat, and look great naked. I was soon to learn that yoga offered much more.

My introduction to yoga came through reading a classic titled *Autobiography of a Yogi*, by Paramahansa Yogananda. I figured anyone with the word "Yoga" in his name must know what he was talking about. Funny thing, the book had nothing to do with stretching and twisting your body into a pretzel. What Yogananda brought to life was a powerful philosophy of living and developing oneself spiritually. I was intrigued, as I had just left ninjutsu and couldn't find another program near my home that inspired me. So the thought that perhaps yoga could fill that void popped into my head after reading the book. The spiritual component was something that I was seeking, even though I was not drawn toward the Hindu mythology glued to the yoga programs I had seen to date. I consider myself a Christian and wondered if there would be a conflict. However, I recalled training at the Zen Mountain Monastery with my karate team back in 1989. The head monk, Daido, said that Buddhism as a philosophy was in complete alignment with Christianity. From what I had read, yoga was similar in that it was not a religion, but a philosophy of living as well and a science of personal development. I thought it could be in complete alignment with any religious conviction. Armed with that theory, my journey into yoga began.

Five years before my deployment to Baghdad I mustered the courage to walk into a Hot Yoga studio in Encinitas, California. In Hot Yoga they crank the temperature up to 105 degrees as you twist and boil your way through 26 poses. The first thing I noticed walking out of the yoga class, dripping wet, was how good I felt. The 90 minutes of standing and seated poses in the sauna-like studio yielded some incredible detoxification and deep-stretching benefits.

Not being one to shy from a gut check, I immediately signed up for their challenge of a Hot Yoga class every day for 60 days. The challenge for me was not so much the discipline, but rather that the classes were chock-full of very attractive women bending and twisting in spandex. Not only was it hard to concentrate, but also my preconditioned notion of what men do and what women do for fitness, was put to the test. I had to trust my intuition that this was a worthy pursuit and shift my attention inward to keep focused on the training effect. I found that this inward focus developed greater awareness and deepened my intuition. It was an experience quite different from my years studying martial arts. In fighting and the martial arts, the focus is mostly outward, except when meditating before and after class. In yoga, it is meant to be inward. Rather than scanning the room or my opponent for opportunities and threats, I was attending to my breathing and the nuances of moving into and staying in the pose. I began to notice that if I went into a session with a scattered mind, the practice settled my mind and connected me to a deeper part of my character.

But Hot Yoga was just a launching pad into this amazing new world. Though a fine introduction to yoga, the precise repeating of the same 26 poses each session, in the same sequence, with the instructors uttering the exact same words each class—became mind-numbing to me. I felt a need for variety and silence in my practice, and I could not get it there. I soon began to wonder if I needed a studio at all. The movements were familiar enough to me after 15 years of martial arts that I thought I would be able to train on my own.

I found two yoga DVDs to use at home. One was by Baron Baptiste, called *Power Yoga* emphasizing core strength and balance, and another by Shiva Rea, emphasizing a fluid, dancelike sequence and breathing. I really enjoyed both as they expanded my repertoire and deepened my knowledge. I would rotate them and add an occasional visit to the Hot Yoga studio to get my sweat on. This went on for 2 years before I stumbled into Ashtanga Yoga, which blew my mind open. Discovering Ashtanga Yoga was a turning point in my yoga studies.

I am lucky to live and work in a town that virtually screams health and fitness. Encinitas, California, brims with world-class endurance athletes, and well-known surfers and skateboarders. Guess what else may be found in Encinitas? Some of the most-qualified yoga teachers in the world. In a conversation with a friend I was asked if I trained with Ashtanga Yoga legend Tim Miller. She said the name with such reverence, she might as well have called him "Master Tim Miller." Tim is the first American to be certified in Ashtanga Yoga by Sri K. Pattabhi Jois. Tim had to train for many years and make several long trips to India, virtually begging Jois for the honor. It was clearly not given out lightly, especially to an American. I found Tim's studio literally across the street from my office. He was the "real deal," and he became my next sensei.

Ashtanga Yoga was derived from the teachings of the famed yoga master Krishnamacharya. He taught Sri K. Pattabhi Jois a progressive system of increasingly challenging series of poses, six series in total, designed for young athletes and military groups. It had a rigid structure that the young men were not to deviate from. After all, good order and discipline are required in the training of new warriors. Jois named it Ashtanga, borrowing the term from Patanjali's Yoga Sutras (more on that in chapter 2). I was drawn to the Ashtanga system because it seemed to share a developmental ladder similar to a martial art belt-ranking system. Though you don't test and get promoted in Ashtanga, you do work progressively through the series of poses over the years. I first approached it with my Western goal-oriented mind, thinking I had found my new martial art and that I was going to "get my black belt in Ashtanga."

My first session of Ashtanga kicked my ass and rekindled the warrior flame within me. It took me—an elite athlete, martial artist, and yoga practitioner—1 hour and 45 minutes to get through, and the session was so demanding I almost lost all bodily functions. I've found the true yoga, I thought with elation, as I crawled off the mat. Later, I would attend two 100-hour teacher trainings in the first and second series with Tim. But as the Iraq War heated up in 2004, duty came knocking again and I replaced my yoga attire with the uniform of the Navy SEALs for the third time.

Welcome to Yoga Saddam

In Baghdad, my yoga session aboard the C-130 stayed with me as I settled into life in the combat zone. My work routine mirrored the "battle rhythm" of the Navy SEAL task group where I set up shop. I would awake around 9:00 a.m. and work till 2:00 or 3:00 a.m. Sleep was a luxury few enjoy in combat.

Exercise was another challenge. SEALs will always improvise to find a way to train, even when operating on combat missions that go late into the night. In my situation it was largely impractical to go to the gym, which was located at Camp Victory and required a combat drive in an armored humvee to get to. It was not worth the risk or time. So I began running around the compound, a 3-mile loop, and doing body weight PT (physical training). Soon I felt the itch for yoga, but there were certainly no yoga classes (that I was aware of) being held anywhere in Baghdad, or Iraq. Another nonstarter. So I again decided to follow my intuition and just go it alone based upon what I had learned from Hot Yoga, Power Yoga, and Ashtanga Yoga.

Finding a small patch near one of Saddam Hussein's former palaces, next to a lake, I set up shop. It wasn't as picturesque as this might sound—for starters, the pool and house were blanketed with pockmarks from a firefight—but it had some trees to provide shade in the desert heat and was removed enough that I wouldn't get awkward stares from the other warriors on base. I skipped breakfast every morning and found refuge at my new training spot. Equipped with a mat, my M4 (now sighted in), and a kettlebell, I started playing with different combinations of yoga poses, functional interval workouts, self-defense moves, and breathing and visualization exercises. The visualization was always of me at home with my family after leaving Baghdad (a version of the "future me" visualization I teach in this book). I would listen closely to my body and train from 45 to 90 minutes depending on what my intuition told me I needed. When I was finished with the practice I felt amazingly clear and calm.

As the weeks progressed this practice became my center post in the storm of combat. One day, CDR Wilson, the commanding officer of SEAL Team 1 stopped by to observe my training. Though he was intrigued, I couldn't get him to join me . . . the demands on his time were simply too much for him to make that leap. Or perhaps he thought what I was doing was a little bit odd, and he didn't want to risk his men thinking I had converted him! I could only explain what it felt like, but a new "initiate" must experience the practice for him or herself to truly understand the vast benefits of yoga. Now, years later, I realize how valuable this practice would be for warriors in the field to manage stress, win in their minds, and avoid the devastating effects of PTSD.

While at the height of the Iraq War, I started each workday feeling calm, energized, in control of my emotions, present, and ready for the mission. My mental facilities were sharp, as were my skills in dealing with the stressful environment. These benefits were, in my opinion, a direct result of the daily yoga practice.

Fast-Forward

My experience in Baghdad was profound and propelled me into taking my life in an entirely new direction. When I returned home I amped up my Ashtanga Yoga practice, and launched US CrossFit and the SEALFIT integrated training program. By 2013 I had a worldwide reputation for success in training SEAL and special ops candidates and other elite athletes through SEALFIT and a mental toughness program called Unbeatable Mind. Based on the training program I wrote three books, two of which became bestsellers. A 20,000-square-foot training center in Encinitas, California, became my laboratory. I could be heard saying, "I eat my own dog food," because I endeavored to train for 2 to 3 hours a day doing a combination of SEALFIT and Kokoro Yoga (and still do to this day).

In 2014, I turned 51 and my body was telling me that I needed to rebalance my training. The combination of the hard-hitting SEALFIT program, with hard-core Ashtanga Yoga, worked well—until I turned 50! Now, it was leading to small injuries and burnout. I needed to find balance in my personal practice, not just for my own comfort, but also so that I could teach athletes and warriors of all ages, not just the younger set. Though I love the Ashtanga practice and community, the rigidity of the routines and difficulty of the poses made me concerned that I would get seriously injured and sidelined as I got older. The warrior's way is to train every day that you are alive, and I planned to be training until 150—then drop dead on the training floor in Savasana (corpse pose!). Thus as I evolved, I wanted my yoga to work for all stages of life, for differing intentions, and for different types of people. A new approach was in order.

I found my next mentor in Gary Kraftsow, founder of American Viniyoga—also adapted from Krishnamacharya's teaching. (Krishnamacharya taught a third application of yoga to B. K. S. Iyengar, which is popular in the West.) These three systems (Ashtanga, Viniyoga, and Iyengar) all seem very different to the observer, but to Krishnamacharya they were just "yoga" taught for different applications and different phases of life. This made sense to me:

In the SEALs we used what worked, discarded what didn't, and strove to adapt our training to our situation, environment, and age. I adopted some Viniyoga training methods so that Kokoro Yoga could be more flexible and balanced.

When asked by my athletes to put my method yoga into a fixed form that could be trained at home or in the field, I was hesitant at first. I always molded it to the audience. And who was I to write a book about yoga in the shadow of such incredible teachers and mentors? But one of my students, a former Marine, asked how his Marines and other military members could train in Kokoro Yoga. He implied that they would be open to try yoga if it came from a warrior like myself, who they trusted to give them practical training to improve their survivability and ability to manage combat-related stress. I received a similar message from my CrossFit "fire-breathing" friend Greg Amundson. He felt that the athletic community needed a yoga that could complement their athleticism through durability, spinal health, and breathing. Finally, I got the blessing from Gary, who felt that this community of warriors desperately needed yoga. I agreed, and this book is my humble attempt to serve.

Whether you are a Navy SEAL running toward the sounds of gunfire or an athlete seeking maximum performance in your sport, a dedicated daily practice of Kokoro Yoga will help you to perform at your peak. If you are suffering from combat (or any shock) related stress, it will allow you to recover your peace of body and mind.

As I found during my time in Baghdad, and have continued to discover to this day, there is incredible value to be absorbed from integrated, full-spectrum training. Do you desire to be more flexible, gain core strength, and be more durable? Yoga will absolutely bring it. Do you want to gain composure under pressure and a calm mind? Yoga will bring it. But that's just the beginning. For the athlete, the military operator, the corporate executive, the artist, the auto mechanic, the firefighter, the student, the homemaker, the parent, I believe Kokoro Yoga is a Trojan horse ready to unleash a host of unforeseen benefits, ultimately leading to the highest levels of consciousness. I know, it sounds too good to be true, but if you stay with me and begin a daily routine that meets your practical needs, body type, and goals, then you will be planting the seeds for a powerful future.

Ultimately, this book is about mastering yourself at all levels so that you can become all you were meant to be. Someone who is willing to say yes to the right mission, and say no to the status quo. Someone who can transcend the various strains of neuroses, which today's media would love to have you feed on, and be "sheepdog strong," so you can serve and protect others. Someone who accelerates their development to the highest, integrated stages of consciousness—and become a world-centric warrior and servant to all of humanity.

CHAPTER 2

THE PURSUIT OF MAXIMUM HUMAN POTENTIAL

When you are inspired by some great purpose, some extraordinary project, all your thoughts break their bonds. Your mind transcends limitations, your consciousness expands in every direction, and you find yourself in a new, great, and wonderful world. Dormant forces, faculties, and talents become alive, and you discover yourself to be a greater person by far than you ever dreamed yourself to be.

—PATANJALI

OLDEST PERSONAL DEVELOPMENT SYSTEM

Just what is yoga? If you think yoga is a group stretching program, or a fitness program for the ladies, then I suggest a visit to northern India to watch how yoga is practiced by the yogi warriors. There you would see how yoga shares its beginnings with the martial traditions, and if you open your mind to fresh understanding of what yoga is, you'll begin to appreciate the depth and breadth of what is the world's oldest and most complete self-development program.

The word *yoga* means "to yoke, to unify, or to integrate." At the mental level it means to integrate your ego mind with your witnessing mind. (Maybe we can call that your soul?) It also means to integrate your body, mind, and spirit into a whole, as well as to live life in a more integrated, balanced manner with simplicity, spirituality, and nonattachment to material distractions. Ultimately I like to focus on yoga as a means to develop mastery of the self, so we can serve others better. We can do this if we integrate fully, connect to our spiritual selves and advance consciousness to the highest level available to us in our lifetime. The word "Kokoro" means warrior spirit, or to merge heart and mind into your actions. So Kokoro Yoga is a warrior development application of this ancient self-realization system.

It's speculated that yoga was first practiced in the fifth or sixth centuries BCE, but it is more plausible that it is thousands of years old. While yoga in the West is most often associated with fitness, or our reverence for Mahatma Gandhi for his yogic philosophy of nonviolent leadership, or Paramahansa Yogananda, founder of the Self-Realization Fellowship, it has a deep, complicated place in India's warrior history in a way that demonstrates the depth and breadth of yoga as a living philosophy of spirituality and science of the mind. As William Pinch detailed in *Warrior Ascetics and Indian Empires*, his account of yoga history in India, he wrote: "Crucial to the transition to wide scale military entrepreneurship in the eighteenth century was the ability of the yogi to be many things at once—to be Muslim and Hindu, emperor and mendicant, ascetic and archer, soldier and spy." Pinch also details the age of India's military labor market and the role yogi warriors or "armed ascetics" had in India's history from 1500 to the present.

Consider the following description of the broad, open-source code nature of yoga by Suketu Mehta, a professor at New York University, who wanted to emphasize how yoga's dimensionality goes beyond fitness or preparing for a fight:

The yoga that most Americans are aware of is Hatha Yoga, only one of the various types of yoga. Krishna in the Bhagavad-Gita defines the others: Raja, Karma, Bhakti,

and Jnana yoga. Yoga is diverse and profound—volunteering at a soup kitchen is yoga; raising your voice in praise in a gospel choir is yoga; trying to understand how the galaxies shift and why the poor lack shoes is also yoga.

The above quote clearly points to yoga being far more than a series of physical movements designed to get you fit and looking good. Jnana Yoga is the yoga of the intellect. Through deep study of scripture, gaining knowledge and wisdom and understanding the working of one's own mind, enlightenment is attained. This is the path many intellectuals in modern religious traditions take. Bhakti Yoga is the path of utter devotion and love for God in a way meaningful to the seeker. This is the path that suits anyone who prefers an "I-Thou" relationship with God. Karma Yoga is the path of action. Through one's dedication to duty and service through action, karma is purified and spiritual evolution occurs. Hatha Yoga is the physical training system for personal mastery that, as Mehta points out, most modern offerings are based upon. In its purest form, Raja Yoga includes Hatha and the study of all eight levels of training described in Patanjali's Yoga Sutras (more on that soon). Where does our yoga fit in this mix?

Kokoro Yoga is designed for anyone who wishes to tap into his or her warrior archetype: those who are driven toward action, passionate about service, and committed to continuous personal growth. It is Raja Yoga that combines Karma Yoga (the yoga of action) with Hatha Yoga (the yoga of personal mastery). We seek to train all of the eight stages of development for self-mastery. As mentioned, these Eight Limbs were defined by Patanjali in the BCE era. Early in my training it was that work that opened my mind to yoga being more than a fitness regimen. I experienced its power as an integrated development system, similar in some ways to what I had experienced with Seido Karate.

THE EIGHT LIMBS

It is said that if you know your enemies and know yourself, you will not be imperiled in a hundred battles; if you do not know your enemies but do know yourself, you will win one and lose one; if you do not know your enemies nor yourself, you will be imperiled in every single battle.—SUN TZU

The Yoga Sutras are a collection of 196 aphorisms (in Sanskrit known as sutras—a thread of specific principles described in terse, cogent pieces of writing). The bulk of the sutras deal with the science of mental development. Yet Patanjali also describes eight levels of the yoga path. They are like rungs on a ladder. The eight levels are to be progressed in a "transcend and include" manner toward a complete integration. This means that each level transcends the level preceding it, but doesn't leave the training and benefits behind. They are included in the upward spiral of development. In sum we are working toward the highest level of integration, which we will call self-mastery. Self-mastery means developing each and every level into a unified whole, so we can experience life at its fullest. Here is a brief description of the Eight Limbs:

LEVEL 1: YAMA. ETHICAL DISCIPLINES. Yama is a code of morality and character to study, align with, and ultimately live by. It can be viewed as a set of ethical disciplines to guide our interactions with other humans. We will discuss some of these disciplines later in the book, and they include a code of restraint, or balance; a code of nonviolence; a code of truthfulness and honesty; a code of nonstealing; a code of noncoveting—meaning the elimination of greed and developing contentment with few possessions and nonindulgence.

LEVEL 2: NIYAMA. PERSONAL DISCIPLINES. These are individual disciplines taken on to set the foundation for mastery of your body and mind, leading to purity and contentment. They include: detoxifying the body and the mind; a deep introspection and healthy use of mental capacities; also, a dedication to a spiritual practice (this can be attending your church, for example). For me, my spiritual practice is yoga and meditation.

LEVEL 3. ASANA. FUNCTIONAL MOVEMENT. This level is what most Westerners think of when they think of yoga. The true purpose of this rung is to prepare the student's body so that he or she can sit in concentration and meditation for long periods of time. For our purposes, this is the movement branch of Kokoro Yoga. It includes the customary poses seen in many yoga studios, and also some functional movements from my SEALFIT program, or CrossFit and even the martial arts.

LEVEL 4. PRANAYAMA. BREATH CONTROL. The fourth level is dedicated to the regulation of breath and harnessing the natural energy all around us. This level is where we begin to transcend from knowing yoga as a physical and ethical practice to experiencing a profound spiritual evolution. Working with the breath is free medicine, bringing optimal health and even great power. Yoga works with prana, or "life force," through the breath. It is identical in this way to practices like Tai Chi (chi meaning "life energy") and Qigong ("life energy cultivation"). Through breath control practices like our box breathing drills, the energy centers of the body are tapped into, linked, and energized through the conscious movement and control of the breath.

LEVEL 5. PRATYAHARA. MASTERY OF THE SENSES. From the extrasensory capacities developed by the deaf and blind, we know that by shutting off one sense, other senses will expand in extraordinary ways to compensate. Thus through level five we seek to train and regulate our senses. By mastering the senses, we can better control those random urges—think about what propels greed and overeating and stuffing our garage with crap we don't really need. By shutting off the senses we can sharpen our capacity to listen to the sixth sense, intuition.

LEVEL 6. DHARANA. CONCENTRATION. This level is about developing deep powers of concentration. We sharpen our mind and develop single-point focus. In practice, this is about brushing away the noise of the unruly mind by strengthening our capacity to lock on to one thing and block out the rest. Martial artists work binding their thoughts, with laserlike focus, to movements. In Kokoro Yoga we will concentrate on the poses, the breath, and an object.

LEVEL 7. DHYANA. MEDITATION. Dhyana is about developing presence. Whereas concentration is a coherent, singular focus, a state of meditation is the absence of thought—settling your witnessing, perceiving mind on the object or subject of your choosing until there is a transfer of information. It is letting go of active thought and being in complete presence. It is at this level of yoga where deep levels of consciousness and awareness are obtained and further trained. In sports, this meditative state is known as flow, or the zone of peak performance, where time stands still and a flow state ensues.

LEVEL 8. SAMADHI. UNION, INTEGRATION. This is considered to be the level of spiritual enlightenment, of the union of true self with the ego self. My friend Ken Wilber, creator of the Integral Theory and author of *The Theory of Everything*, explains that when integrated ("enlightened" in Eastern terminology) you will tether with your "soul self" which then becomes the center of your consciousness versus your limited ego-thinking self. When this happens we end separation and are able to express ourselves most authentically to the world, able to take perspectives on our own perspectives as well as those of others, and can experience life as a blissful connection with all sentient beings.

HISTORICAL INFLUENCES

Now that you have a sense of the depth and breadth of yoga, let's get a grasp of the historical roots. However, considering the hundreds or thousands of years that yoga has existed, a definitive history of yoga is beyond the capacity of this book. What I do wish to impart is that yoga has had many expressions and can be considered an open-source project taken on by warriors, athletes, and spiritual aspirants over many eons. The project continues today with millions of Western practitioners adopting its methods and philosophy.

Arjuna: A Warrior at a Crossroads

The mind is restless, turbulent, strong and unyielding . . . as difficult to subdue as the wind. For the uncontrolled there is no wisdom. Nor for the uncontrolled is there power of concentration. And for him without concentration there is no peace. And for the unpeaceful how can there be happiness—ADAPTED FROM THE *BHAGAVAD GITA* (KRISHNA SPEAKING TO ARJUNA)

A text that routinely appears in comparative religion classes throughout the Western world is the *Bhagavad Gita*. The Hindu epic, composed circa the seventh century BCE, presented the many faces of yoga and how they appeal to certain characters such as the warrior Arjuna. A central theme is the importance of performing one's simple, daily work and duties with a critical and spiritual binding with renunciation—of not being attached to material rewards. The *Gita* is a warrior's manual that encourages the reader to actively confront and take on evil in the world rather than turning the other cheek.

At the heart of the *Gita* is a dialogue between Arjuna, a master archer warrior, and Krishna, an earthly manifestation of the Indian deity Vishnu, representing the voice of God. A major battle is about to erupt between Arjuna's tribe and his cousin's tribe. Arjuna is confronted with the fact that his mission requires fighting against members of his family—the sort of inner conflict that Americans recall from their history of the Civil War. Arjuna's skill with the bow and arrow is so exceptional that he can pierce the eye of a bird in flight, but in the *Gita* he struggles with questions of morality, ethics, and his duty as a warrior, seeking answers from Krishna. Arjuna ultimately chooses not to fight, sacrificing his life rather than betray his thoughts and feelings for his family. The dialogue with Krishna finally offers a path to spiritual freedom that is not total renunciation of the fruits of one's labor nor abstinence from performing one's work—rather, spiritual perfection is pursued by performing one's duty in life without looking for rewards and with detachment to the results. Arjuna's sacrifice informs the inner struggle of warriors of all races and generations, including the modern warrior who strives to do the right thing in spite of the consequences.

Bodhidharma and Kalaripayattu

In surveying the expansion of yoga from the ancient East to the modern West, we should also look at the shared roots yoga has with the martial arts. The legend of Bodhidharma, a son of an Indian King in the sixth century, sheds light on both of these topics. Bodhidharma traveled by foot and boat from his homeland, where he eventually arrived at the Shaolin Monastery in the Henan Province of China, the famous Buddhist temple known for the development of Kung Fu. Martial arts history holds that after Bodhidharma arrived at the temple, he spent 9 years in seated meditation, inspiring the monks with both his fierce discipline and deep spiritual powers. Bodhidharma began to teach the monks the practice of what would be known as Zen meditation, but the monks were academics and didn't have the physical capacities to perform extended meditation.

Bodhidharma created what you might call a health and fitness program to complement the meditation practice, a series of 18 flowing yoga postures very similar to Hatha Yoga. The movements also shared properties of the Indian martial art known as Kalaripayattu—which is considered by some to be the oldest fighting art in human history. Bodhidharma has been credited by some for the creation of Shaolin Boxing and his contribution to Zen Buddhism. There is ample evidence that the Chinese had developed martial systems far before Bodhidharma arrived, but the key point I'd like to make is that through this form of educational dissemination, the ancient practice of yoga was transmitted across borders and eventually throughout the world.

Yoga and Gymnastics

In sorting out the modern offerings of yoga in the West, it can be helpful to reverse engineer the influences and reinterpretations involved. One of the more interesting discussions, sparked by author Mark Singleton, suggests that there was a blending of West into East as modern yoga evolved. Singleton's book, *Yoga Body,* pins some of his research on a fitness trend that occurred in Europe in the nineteenth century. It was then that the Scandinavian system of gymnastics became popular throughout Europe in the 1800s. Called "primitive gymnastics"—and showing up in the YMCA network of gymnasiums—it was a bodyweight exercise regimen, attractive to civilians for the health benefits and attractive to the fighting forces for the fitness edge it could provide. The poses used within the Danish system are vividly similar to the poses you'd find in an introduction to yoga class.

Following is an interesting assessment by writer Matthew Lee Anderson on the *Yoga Body*:

> Mark Singleton analyzed Niels Bukh's *Primary Gymnastics* (1925) and found that "at least 28 of the exercises in the first edition of Bukh's manual are strikingly similar (often identical) to yoga postures occurring in Pattabhi Jois' Ashtanga sequence or in Iyengar's *Light on Yoga*. Both Jois and Iyengar were students of T. Krishnamacharya, who taught yoga in the Indian royal palace and whose classes were categorized as "physical culture" or "exercise" in the official palace records. By that point, the Danish gymnastic system had reached such a level of popularity that it had been incorporated into the British Army and into the Indian YMCA.

Yoga Comes to American Shores

The European explosion of yoga and gymnastics for exercise was a precursor to several key yoga voices crossing the pond to introduce Americans to the mysteries of yoga. One of the most influential was Paramahansa Yogananda, from Uttar Pradesh, India, who came to the United States in 1920. Through Yogananda's establishment of the Self-Realization Fellowship and his book, *Autobiography of a Yogi* (incidentally this is the only book Steve Jobs kept on his personal iPad), he introduced the philosophy of yoga, and meditation to millions. Other teachers that have had a big impact on the popularity of yoga in the United States include

Mr. Universe winner Walt Baptiste, followed by his son Baron. Baron has more recently popularized Power Yoga, a variant of Ashtanga Vinyasa (flowing) Yoga. With Power Yoga he weaves mind-and-body empowerment practice including meditation and "active self-enquiry." Baron became a performance coach for the Philadelphia Eagles, an early pioneer in applying yoga methods for sports performance.

Yoga continues to evolve to this day. As Kaitlin Quistgaard, former editor-in-chief of *Yoga Journal*, put it: "With around 15 million Americans practicing yoga, there's room for diversity and for the practice to evolve in more than one direction at a time."

PERFORM LIKE A MASTER

One of the chief purposes of this book is to make a cogent case for why an integrated somatic practice like Kokoro Yoga can serve up profound performance improvements for first responders, military operators, CrossFitters, endurance athletes, and, frankly, anyone committed to self-mastery in the service of others. The path of Kokoro Yoga is to blend physical, mental, emotional, intuitive, and spiritual training to positively impact performance on the playing field, peace of mind in the battle zone, presence in a boardroom, and fitness while on the road.

So what does peak performance look like in a flow state?

The quarterback sizzling first-down strikes in a championship game—his eyes pierced in concentration, as if in another universe altogether—relaxed and oblivious to the crowd noise and the millions watching on TV; the SEAL team silently executing the Bin Laden raid in cool, fluid precision despite the stress and chaos of the combat zone; the CrossFitter in a fury during the workout of the day (WOD) as she continues to execute pull-ups and thrusters with power and grace, despite the onslaught of pain and fatigue cooking within the muscles and through her lungs. These are just a few examples of the connection between states of mind and performance, where it's abundantly clear that mental preparation, mental toughness, and accessing flow figure into physical performance capacity.

This door swings both ways: As 2013 World Chess Champion Viswanathan Anand said in an interview with *Complete Well Being,* "In chess, since we have to prepare for about 7–8 hours [of competition] a day, physical fitness is as essential as mental fitness." He added that emotional control also figures into the nature of the peak performance state. "For me, as it is for everyone, feelings determine performance," he said. "Only when you are happy or feel good about yourself can you play well. I try to keep my life simple, as chess itself is very complicated." So, according to the chess master, physical, mental, and emotional aspects all play into peak performance.

In other words, to generate and maintain top performance, we must supercharge the physical with mental and the emotional aspects of training. This is true whether you are training to be a chess master, a Navy SEAL, or an elite corporate warrior. Another compelling example from the world stage is Japan's Ichiro Suzuki, Major League Baseball's ten-time All-Star. Here are a few details about Ichiro's integrated approach to his sport:

Ichiro Suzuki painstakingly cleans every piece of his equipment, including shoes and glove, before each game. He has done this for 22 seasons, during an amazing career that has stretched across two continents. He keeps his bats in a humidor-like carrying case.

His physical preparation is just as thorough. He begins his gameday routine with weight lifting and a series of stretching exercises and yoga-like poses . . . After games, he records his thoughts on the day in a personal journal.—RICHARD JUSTICE, "MODEL OF EXCELLENCE: ICHIRO REACHES 4,000 HITS HIS WAY," MLB.COM

And this from another source:

When he gazed in the general direction of the crowd he was staring a hole right through us. He was totally locked in. He was in a place far away, some sort of deep font of performance excellence.—JUSTIN PANSON, "ICHIRO, WHAT IS THE MEANING OF LIFE?" CONFLUENCE STUDIO

What Ichiro has is what I call an unfettered mind, which comes from a special form of training. I call that training integrated warrior development. This program is a structured version of such a regimen, in that it integrates the mental, emotional, physical, and spiritual intelligences to prepare for "battle," similar to how Ichiro did in his training.

TRAIN FOR LIFE

Maybe it is abundantly clear by now that Kokoro Yoga is more than a workout. It is training that can meet you where you are at, and stay with you for life. You will change the methods to suit your needs over time. Which poses, functional exercises, sequences, breathing, concentration, and visualization drills you use will depend upon your age, body type, season of the year, and intentions. My hope is also that you appreciate that the training is presented from a Western warrior's point of view. The language is familiar and avoids cultural nuances found in most other yoga training—such as the Sanskrit pose names, Hindu mythology, and chanting. The following core principles define the full experience of our system, each of which will be explored in greater detailed later in this book:

BOTH A PRACTICE AND A LIFESTYLE: Kokoro Yoga can be both a practice, providing powerful tools to aid in your physical and mental training, as well as a set of principles for living an enriched, unbeatable life.

FLEXIBLE AND VARIABLE: Variety is the spice of life and Kokoro Yoga is flexible, providing for maximum variability to meet your specific needs. Doing the same rigidly fixed form year in and year out will lead to a rut, burnout, and injury. Variety is a good thing and can be found by changing up pose sequences for a particular effect, changing the duration based on your time and intention, and also flexing your practice into the times of the day that you train. While taking a modular approach to the practice allows for maximum variety and learning, it can also lead to avoiding things that are challenging and could help you break through to a new level. You will explore this concept as your practice evolves.

INTENTIONAL: Rather than just hitting a yoga class for a workout, we are clear about the intention for our training, and the desired result for each session. For instance, using the Hip Mobility Drill after a CrossFit WOD is intended to open the hips, develop flexibility and durability, calm the nervous system after ramping it up, and immediately trigger the recovery process. Doing a session in the morning when you wake up is intended to facilitate spinal health, stimulate your nervous system, clear your mind, and charge you positively to provide a foundation of excellence for your day. Kokoro Yoga can be performed to enhance athleticism, to develop strong leadership traits, and for spiritual enlightenment. In the case of a warrior, all of these goals are relevant and will be developed with the methods employed in these pages.

BALANCED: Train hard, train soft. Train long, train short. We use yoga to find balance in our bodies, minds, and lives. We seek a balance between effort and surrender, between work and recovery. If you have a bone-crushing CrossFit workout, then you would do a moderate restorative yoga session to balance the effort and energy of the workout.

However, if you are on vacation and yoga is your primary training, due to space and time constraints (which is often my case), then balance may mean including a bodyweight WOD module into an hour-long challenging session (see the Fit Warrior sequence in chapter 5) . . . similar to how I trained in Baghdad.

ADAPTABLE: We adapt the pose to our bodies rather than try to adapt our body to the pose. I learned this by contrasting how Ashtanga Yoga is taught versus Viniyoga. In Ashtanga the pose is the pose, and you exert extreme effort to contort your body to the pose structure. This approach, if performed unwisely or when not prepared, can lead to injury. In Viniyoga, the approach is to move into the pose with repetitions to refine the functional movement pattern, and then to stay in the full expression of the pose that is appropriate for you in that moment. We have adopted this sensible model for Kokoro Yoga, where you approach a pose with your own level of flexibility, mobility, functional fitness, and prior injuries that you need to adapt for. Even the time of day and season of the year will influence how our bodies and minds react to a pose, and how we should wisely approach it.

INTEGRATED: Already discussed at length, our premise is that accelerated growth occurs when we embody training in an integrated manner. You will be developing yourself physically, mentally, morally, emotionally, intuitionally, and spiritually. These intelligences are deeply connected and when you actively integrate the training of them they will conspire to unlock your full potential as a human.

FIXED AND FLOWING: We use an approach that embraces both static form and flowing movement. What I mean by this is that we will do some poses with no flow, and others we will flow with the breath between poses, but then stay in some poses for a fixed amount of time or breath cycles to allow our bodies to sink deeper into the pose. This allows for a deepening of concentration and awareness. In addition, there are some flowing poses that are mostly about the breathing technique that has a particular effect on your body or mind. These poses look more like Tai Chi than traditional yoga. Keep in mind that yoga, in its original form thousands of years ago, was a warrior and spiritual development training method that has deep connections with Tai Chi, Qigong, and other martial arts as it spread west from India into Tibet and regions now known as China, Korea, and Japan.

THE RESULTS

Indeed, Kokoro Yoga is designed to do far more for you than help you work up a sweat. It is about developing a warrior spirit, merging your heart and mind into your actions so you can achieve your maximum human potential. In the next chapter, we'll take a thorough look at the strategies that allow for the integration of the training to work its magic.

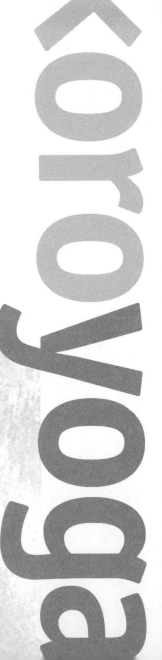

CHAPTER 3

THE STRATEGIES

Happiness is when what you think, what you say, and what you do are in harmony.

—MAHATMA GANDHI

NAVY SEALS RELY ON BOTH STRATEGIES AND TACTICS TO ACCOMPLISH THEIR MISSION. STRATEGIES ARE THE OVERARCHING METHODS EMPLOYED TO DIRECT THE ENERGIES, FOCUS, AND RESOURCES OF THE TEAM. TACTICS ARE THE SPECIFIC METHODS THE TEAMS WILL EMPLOY TO GET THE ACTUAL JOB DONE. IN THIS CHAPTER I WANT TO SPEND TIME NOW ON THE CORE STRATEGIES WITHIN THE KOKORO YOGA PROGRAM—WHY WE DO THINGS A CERTAIN WAY. YOU'LL NOTICE THAT the strategies are linked to the wisdom of the original Eight Limbs of yoga, informed through my personal experience training thousands of modern-day warriors since 2007. With an understanding of the strategic engines firmly established, we'll then take a look at the ground-level tactics in chapter 4: the nuts, bolts, and basic methods of how we execute these strategies.

STRATEGY 1: DEVELOP A PERSONAL ETHOS

Excellence outcomes in life are built upon a personal philosophy, or code, of excellence. I call this a personal ethos. Defining this ethos requires deep introspection and skillful methods leading to a continuous pursuit of self-knowledge and growth. Training without a personal ethos can leave you directionless, not able to answer the question, *Why?*, when faced with life's many challenges.

"The mass of men lead lives of quiet desperation," wrote Henry David Thoreau, exposing a truth that holds true today. Finding stillness to eliminate the noise and distractions that obscure the voice of our soul from being heard is not easy, but crucial for us to find and fulfill our purpose. Rather than reacting like a pinball to the myriad of forces and stressors rushing at us every day, we must take time to question deeply what we are meant for, what we are passionate about, and how we can serve meaningfully through our unique gifts.

We must question what societal and family beliefs make the best fit, and begin to orient ourselves to universal laws and positive (love) energy so that we can allow our uniqueness and beauty to flow out of us like a river. We start this process by asking deep questions, working to separate from ego identification with our roles, challenges, issues, and obsessions. As we gain clarity on the Yamas and Niyamas introduced in the last chapter, we connect deeper with our witnessing self, your "soul self." In deep connection with your witness you are said to act from your "True Self" as opposed to your "False Self," which is guided by your ego.

A good place to enact your code of conduct is to examine and align with the five precepts called Yamas, that lead the way to excellence and are a contemplation as well as an ethical practice. Aligning with these precepts will produce a profound grounding effect on your life. These are codes of restraint and self-regulations that have us acknowledge our interconnected relationship with all sentient beings and the environment, and to align with them in a spirit of harmony. They are:

1. Nonviolence to oneself or others. This code of conduct poses a challenge for warriors. Keep in mind that duty plays a role, as Arjuna learned.

2. Speaking, thinking, and acting truth.

3. Not hoarding unnecessarily. Being honest with what belongs to you, what belongs to others, and what belongs to the common good.

4. Balancing your energy in work, play, and relationships.

5. Not grasping for or getting attached or clinging to ideas, material objects, or relationships.

These five precepts, when asked as questions, provide a powerful guide for our actions and thoughts. Establishing a code that is grounded with these five precepts will lead to a balanced and positive relationship with all stakeholders in the great web of life. The code in action is your integrity. They are to be practiced in thoughts, words, and deeds. Becoming aware of how you live the precepts is important. How do you act truthful? How do you speak truthfully? How do you think of truth? Truth is different in the domains of action, speech, and thought. To have integrity means they are aligned.

We next want to examine and refine our habits or Niyamas, which ground the journey toward personal mastery. These are:

■ Developing purity and control of the body and mind. We accomplish this with proper fueling and a daily practice of functional fitness and asana, or some other skillfully executed method of somatic movement training.

■ Contentment of one's circumstances in life. We are where we are for a reason, so be okay with it while working methodically to improve your own condition and the condition of the world . . . one relationship at a time.

■ Taking control over your desires, the constant grasping at pleasure and striving to avoid pain. Neither pleasure nor pain is good or bad on its own, but it is the craving or avoidance that makes it so. Consider the avoidance of the pain associated with intense physical training. Choosing to avoid this kind of temporary discomfort means that we won't develop our warrior body and mind. Or being constantly drawn to the pleasure of sweets. Consistently folding to this weakness means that we sacrifice control and we slowly kill ourselves with sugar.

- **Self study and study of sacred texts.** This is one aspect of the deeply spiritual component of yoga. It's about what we choose to focus our mind upon, whether our internal states of mind and emotion, or a parable of Jesus, we come to understand deeply. Our awareness of reality and knowledge of the nature of things increases.

- **Surrender to a higher power.** This is your concept of God, whether you have a religious orientation or not. If not, Gaia, the Tao, or "Spirit that runs through all things" will do just fine. Let go of the mental grasping and contracting of ego self, and surrender to a "now" presence where you can connect to this power. This practice will lead to more energy and keep you in alignment with your True Self.

The discipline habits are meant to tame the body, mind, and senses so that we can advance our training through concentrated study and meditation. Similar to the first five precepts, they characteristically arise in thought, speech, and action as if there were three elements of practice needing to be trained together. For instance, do you think you are content? Do you talk about contentment and do you act content? Upon deep reflection you may find that there are subtle differences in each of these, and this awareness leads you to work toward their alignment.

Write down any insights that come to you as you consider your relationship to the above precepts and disciplines. Review them weekly and note what comes up in your silence practices. You will be developing a powerful personal ethos through this process. Ultimately you want to always be able to answer the following questions: Why am I doing this? Why is this happening to me? Am I aligned with my ethos?

This level of self-study naturally draws us even deeper inward, to places we previously didn't know existed. This is where we must travel to and spend time exploring the root answer of the questions about your reality. When you can answer the question, Why?, you can better answer the questions: What am I going to do about this? How and with whom? Of course at the heart of these questions lies the one question that is the very essence of what it means to be human:

Who am I?

Taking time to settle into these ponderous issues is the next step in the awakening process of the first strategy. These are questions stoked with power; leave them unasked, or unanswered, and you're sure to drift along as I did in the first 24 years of my life. Asking them, and reflecting on what comes up in silence, will slowly but definitely lead to the construction of a deep personal ethos. As daunting as this may seem, I want you to know how rewarding and dynamic this process is, and how it opens you up like a flower awakening to the dawn. The answers you have to these questions today will evolve over time as you continue to work the program. They will inform the choices you make, the projects you take on, and the values you establish. You will cultivate honor and integrity as you align your actions with your growing sense of ethos and purpose in life. As you become more comfortable with this insight work you will gain the traction and energy that comes from clarifying your identity and knowing what you stand for.

The development of your personal ethos counts on silence to be your guide. We plant the questions in our minds and trust the daily rituals to draw answers up from the depths, as if through a magnetic force. New insights about the questions and deeper awareness will bubble to the surface and reveal themselves as insights, new ideas, feelings, or images.

The following are the core questions to ask before your practice sessions, particularly the morning and evening rituals (discussed in chapter 8):

Who am I?

Why am I here—what is my purpose?

What unique passion can I offer the world?

What and whom do I love?

Am I positive and helpful?

How can I boldly serve my family, team, country, world?

What do I value and want to bring more of into my life?

What do I want less of in my life?

A great example of a morning ritual would be to ask these questions and follow with box breathing, a short yoga sequence, and then to meditate on aligning your personal ethos with Yamas and Niyamas. Over time you will be able to articulate the answers to the above questions clearly. You will know beyond a shadow of a doubt just who you are right now, where you're at in your life, and where you need to go. It's from this rich material that you will build your powerful and driving vision for your life. This first strategy of developing a personal ethos is critical to living the warrior's way, so don't shortcut it or think you already have all the answers. Humility is to admit that you do not know everything . . . and in fact, the more you learn, the less you seem to know about the mysteries of the world! Now on to the next strategy: to develop body awareness, control, and optimal physical health.

STRATEGY 2: FUNCTIONAL CONDITIONING

The second strategy is to optimize your functional movement capacity. We do this with classic "asana" poses intelligently sequenced, as well as with mindfully performed functional exercises. One of the paradigm shifts we've seen in the last decade has been an embrace of functional fitness. In Kokoro Yoga, we rely on traditional poses of yoga—those you see in any yoga class. But we also rely on functional movements of CrossFit and SEALFIT to close gaps, or weaknesses, in physical conditioning found in other yoga systems. This does not mean you have to become a CrossFit or SEALFIT athlete to do this program. The movements are simple and scalable for all practitioners. It simply means that this yoga could be your complete integrated training system for both "working out" and "working in." Functional movements are comprised of exercises that involve compound movements and universal motor recruitment patterns—like push-ups, burpees, and squats—as opposed to traditional gym equipment. The term "universal" refers to the natural use of full-body patterns that mimic physical movements in our daily lives, such as digging a ditch, shoveling snow, hiking in rugged terrain, and chopping wood.

The conditioning modules we present get quick results by performing functional movements with high-intensity, building cardiovascular endurance, strength, stamina, and power. This work also leads to deep awareness of the body and greater confidence in the performance of work and play outdoors.

The functional movements we depend upon for the Fit Warrior and Protective Warrior sequences are classic body-weight gymnastics and "cardio-kickboxing" movements. Having said that, on occasion kettlebells, dumbbells, or sand bags can be utilized to augment the impact of the training. The work is performed in the context of the yoga sequence as an embedded module. Doing the yoga then going to the gym is old school. If you do not have a functional fitness regimen at the moment, then this program will get you on your way by performing three rigorous sessions a week, using Fit Warrior and Protective Warrior sequences. This program will deliver excellent functional fitness and health, all geared toward supporting you on that journey to excellence.

FIVE LAYERS OF BEING

Before moving on to the next strategy, this is a good place to insert some comments about the five dimensions of the self. These were called the "pancamayas" (five pervasive layers) in the ancient Vedic text Taittiriya Upanishad wherein the Rishis introduced ancient yoga philosophy to the world. These dimensions are aspects of our being to access, align, and develop in a holographic manner through the science of yoga. Modern science is making progress understanding the first three, but lacks credible means to penetrate the latter two, which are the realm of deep interior development.

THE PHYSICAL DIMENSION

The outermost of the layers is literally called the food layer by the ancient yogis. This layer is built by food and can become food if we find ourselves in the jungle alone. It is the aspect of our beings that is trained with the second strategy of Kokoro Yoga, functional movement. But it also requires effective fueling and sleeping habits for the care of and nurturing of the body to allow us to fulfill our purpose and live in happiness. When we take care of the physical being we are able to journey inward without our bodies being distracted with pain, injuries, or disease, such as when we sit in meditation. The physical body has been the focus of Western fitness, but has lacked much acknowledgment of the other layers. In Kokoro Yoga we strive to train and develop all layers simultaneously for optimal effect.

ENERGETIC DIMENSION

The next dimension is the vital, energetic layer. This is the vital force that turns the lights on in our human house. The energy is produced internally through metabolism, and is also brought in from the outside through the breath, thoughts, and our environment. Kokoro Yoga seeks to refine and train this level of our being for optimal energy flow through pathways in the body called Nadis. Through Pranayama, or breath control training (i.e., box breathing), we get intimate with the energy body, explore it, and roam further inward to additional layers.

MENTAL DIMENSION

The next dimension is the mental. This level is for cognizing, learning, and learning how to learn. In this dimension we take in information from our senses, process it as thoughts and emotions, and then seek meaning in the world. The mental aspect of our being is the judger, feeler, and supervisor of our lives. In modern terms this would be the rational mind, centered in the neocortex. The mental being is tuned to sniff for danger and opportunities (in fact all inbound information is initially processed through the amygdala, the main purpose of which is to discriminate between things to fear and not fear).

Negativity can prevail in the mental layer with obsessive, negative associations and weak thinking—a disease of our modern world. Through the practice of Kokoro Yoga we strive to gain control over this crucial dimension, train it to be positive and uncovering truth, then to connect with the next dimension, the wisdom of personality. As this happens the mind is cleared of doubt and illusion and we can connect with our true self—that aspect of your mind that receives clear reflection of reality from deep wisdom. A fully developed mental dimension allows us then to express our uniqueness fully, uncluttered by fear or deception.

WISDOM DIMENSION

The next is the wisdom dimension, that aspect of our being that can discern an innate, felt knowingness of purpose and drives your deeper, "true self," or authentic, personality. Excessive thinking in the mental dimension can get in the way of accessing this wisdom layer. The deep wisdom that lies in all of us and is found by cultivating sacred silence. This dimension is felt in our heart and belly regions and discriminates between good and bad, useful and not useful. Deep conditioning, patterns, and habits are grooved into this layer over this lifetime, and possibly even past lives.

When accessed, the wisdom dimension brings us into deep connection to others, all of humanity and the earth. The sensations from this layer are beyond thoughts—and are always positive. The wisdom dimension is "the courage wolf" that lies within us, that generator of love in all of its forms. Through our integrated training we can connect with our wisdom, dimensions, eradicate negative patterns, and uncover the love that lies within. Then we are empowered to go even deeper within, in search of the eternal center of bliss consciousness.

BLISS DIMENSION

The bliss dimension is the most interior of the layers and it connects to the seat of consciousness itself. When connected to, this layer is experienced as radical bliss, peace, and joy beyond the mind, independent of any stimulus that may trigger a happy or blissful mental reaction. In short, it is your capacity for happiness without any extrinsic reason for being happy. The ancient yogis said that the bliss experienced as this dimension is accessed is 1,000 times more powerful than the highest form of mentally experienced joy. Wow.

In the silence of deep meditation, in service to others, and in moments of total presence in a purposeful, passionate pursuit, this bliss is released. We are experiencing a connection to the center of our soul. Hard to put into words, but it is called different names by various traditions (i.e., Atman, Christ Consciousness). It is our eternal center that was never born and never dies. Accessing the bliss dimension is the direct experience of a long-term integration practice and it will unlock our full potential as it allows our unique beauty to express itself fully.

STRATEGY 3: MENTAL AND EMOTIONAL CONTROL

The second Sutra of Patanjali is "yogah citta vrtti nirodah." This means that yoga (integration) comes from the ability to concentrate the mind until all thoughts are under one's control. Then we can direct the mind exclusively toward an object or subject and sustain that without any distractions for as long as desired. This speaks to the power of yoga for forging mental and emotional control. If we consider that emotions are primal and stored thoughts experienced not as words in our heads, but as feelings in our bodies, then we can surmise that Patanjali included emotional control in this definition.

One of the defining qualities of being human is our gift to experience feelings that lead to meaning. This doesn't happen by just thinking something over: rather, it's the connection between real experiences, the thoughts that come with those experiences, and the emotions provoked by those thoughts. This is the space where we have an opportunity to cultivate deep learning and connection. It is also the most overlooked and undertrained area of development for many of us.

Thoughts and emotions are part of the mental dimension. Through concentration, meditation, and visualization practice we seek to manage our mental and emotional selves so we can direct thoughts and emotions positively and intentionally toward fulfilling our personal ethos. An example is how we deal with fear. When we experience fear such as with a life-threatening situation, through our training we learn to face the fear and transmute the mental and emotional energy of it into a more positive and focused energy (such as determination), which will help to survive and end the threat. Navy SEALs are modern yoga practitioners in that they are masters at this form of mental and emotional management.

In this strategy we seek a level of control over our lives that is uncommon in our busy, modern world. Your concentration, focus, and overall awareness will improve as a result of the daily practice of the integrated training. With this deeper connection you will have at your command greater control to detect and direct your thoughts and emotions in a purpose-filled direction.

STRATEGY 4: BREATH MASTERY

I learned during my SEAL training just how powerful mastery of the breath could be. I am confident that this one strategy led to my big success there, and later as a Special Ops and business leader. It is now the first thing I teach to aspiring Navy SEAL candidates at SEALFIT.

Breathing is a unique system in the human body; unlike, for example, digestion, breathing has both an involuntary control mechanism as well as voluntary, similar to a 747 in that it can shift between being piloted and being left on autopilot. If you are a military special operator, or have a background with martial arts or yoga, it's likely that you inherently understand the strategy of mastering the breath. If not, you will find the most immediate practical benefits in your life from this strategy. When you begin the box breathing practice you will note an immediate impact in the form of lower stress, a heightened, alert focus, and a calmer mind. Strategy 4 strives to accomplish the following three aims:

1. First, air is our primary source of fuel so learning how to get the most out of each "bite" can lead to many health and longevity benefits (see chapter 7 for more on the benefits). Most people are unaware of this simple truth, as well as of their own breathing patterns. The average person is accustomed to panting some 25,000 shallow breaths throughout the day, or 16 to 20 breaths per minute. If this is you, then you should know that in doing so you are using just a fraction of the natural lung capacity you are born with, and you are keeping your body in a constant state of agitation in the process.

2. Controlling the breath controls our stress, or fight, flight, or freeze response. Shallow, choppy, and irregular chest breathing stimulates the fight-or-flight, sympathetic nervous system, ratcheting up urgency and stress. A calm, deep, and measured belly breath, on the other hand, stimulates the rest and digest, parasympathetic system, dialing down stress, slowing the heart rate, and calming the entire body down.

3. Breath control is a bridge to mental control. When I learned as a martial artist to control my breathing during intense fighting bouts it proved invaluable later during the chaos of combat. As noted above I found that it both calmed my body and mind—bringing them immediately under control, allowing me to focus on my targets and make good decisions.

To help achieve these aims, you'll be performing breath control exercises in the training sessions. These exercises will link breath to the movements. You will note in the sequencing that we specify when to breathe in and out, so that you ride the breath like a surfer riding a long wave. Over time you will cultivate greater energy, the same energy that martial artists refer to as "chi" and yogis refer to as "prana." We will get into the practical steps for mastering the breath in the next chapter on tactics.

STRATEGY 5: SENSE MASTERY

When I trained in the martial art of ninjutsu, I spent a lot of time developing what we called sensual awareness. No—it wasn't so we could be better in bed (though it didn't hurt). Rather this was about developing the sense "doors" by opening them to receive more information. Through this training I became more nuanced in interpreting the received information and making more sense out of it. Was that tingling sensation a signal of danger? Was the ripple in energy someone entering the room, disrupting my energy matrix? Many warriors who have seen combat have experienced enhanced sensory awareness as an adaptation to the risk.

However, when the warriors get back to "normal life" they note that those sense doors seem to close again. I believe that we can train to keep these doors open so that our intuition is always clear and accessible—allowing us to make better decisions and be more effective warriors and leaders.

In performing the poses and flowing between poses, you are meant to focus your mind and senses inward. For example, you'll want to tune down your sense of hearing and narrow your sight to a single-point focus. Or you will soften your gaze or close your eyes altogether and focus on the sound of your breathing. Or perhaps you will let your inner awareness rest on a point in the body, such as a joint, muscle, or energy center (cakra). Intuition, as intelligence, is not experienced verbally, but sensationally and via imagery. Therefore, within this work of mastering the senses, we will be developing the language of imagery and sensations, rather than words. This is difficult to convey in a book, of course. It is your job to constantly scan your body for sensations, insights, and images from your intuition. Turning the senses inward during practice helps us to tune and expand the senses more fully for our overall awareness of the nature of self, others, and the world.

STRATEGY 6: INTEGRATION

The above five strategies work together toward supporting the final strategy that I call integration. Kokoro Yoga drives toward achieving an integration and union of the five dimensions as well as our True Self with our clarified egoic self. But what does this integration feel like? At the external "service" level it is experienced as effortless success, meaning that the entire world seems to conspire to support your mission and purpose in life. At the internal "self-mastery" level it is experienced as a world-centric consciousness, peaceful and mastery over your mind and emotions. The Japanese concept of *shibumi,* "effortless perfection," is a nice way to express this experience. You will effortlessly perfect your trade or art, as you are meant to with your unique and innate skills and talents, and in doing so you will find great joy in your work.

Integration allows you to unlock a flow state at will. When I train this with long-term coaching clients the process is greatly accelerated due to the intensity and enmeshment of all the senses in the training. Students learn how to turn on and off flow through the big four skills of breath control, positivity, visualization, and micro-goals. Flow is the psychological term coined by Mihaly Csikszentmihalyi, a psychology professor at the University of Chicago and author of *Flow: The Psychology of Optimal Experience.* In his book, Csikszentmihalyi defines this flow as a state of absorption with the moment and with what one is doing, and he makes an acute comparison to yoga: "The similarities between [integration in] yoga and flow are extremely strong; in fact it makes sense to think of yoga as a very thoroughly planned flow activity. Both try to achieve a joyous, self-forgetful involvement through concentration, which in turn is made possible by a discipline of the body."[1]

As he later said to *Wired* magazine, "The ego falls away. Time flies. Every action, movement, and thought follows inevitably from the previous one, like playing jazz. Your whole being is involved, and you're using your skills to the utmost."

Csikszentmihalyi notes that the relationship between the difficulty of a task we take on, and our training or experience in performing said task, impacts our ability to remain present and access flow. The ideal is to have the challenge slightly greater than our training level—so pushing the envelope with training, then pushing the envelope performing, has a positive upward spiral effect on performance, at both a personal and team level, because it creates the conditions for flow to "present" itself.

Steven Kotler writes in his book, *The Rise of Superman,* that there are also several environmental, psychological, social, and creative triggers for flow to occur. Deep embodiment is one of the environmental triggers. That means being able to pay attention to

---

[1]Mihaly Csikszentmihalyi, *Flow: The Psychology of Optimal Experience* (New York: Harper & Row, 1990), 105.

multiple sensory inputs simultaneously. Time becomes relative—there is no concept of past or future that might otherwise be dogging us in the form of regret or worry.

Now, with these six overarching strategies in mind, I'd like to run through the tactics in the next chapter—the essential tools and techniques you'll be employing to effectively train with this program.

CHAPTER 4

THE TACTICS

A gem cannot be polished without friction, nor a man perfected without trials.

—CHINESE PROVERB

WHEREAS A STRATEGY IS A HIGH-LEVEL ORIENTATION OR PLAN FOR HOW TO ACCOMPLISH A MISSION, A TACTIC IS A GROUND-LEVEL METHOD, TECHNIQUE, OR PROCEDURE FOR MOVING THE DIAL IN THE CHOSEN STRATEGIC DIRECTION. FOR INSTANCE, IN SPECIAL OPERATIONS THE STRATEGY WOULD BE TO USE SPEED TO SURPRISE THE ENEMY. A TACTIC THE SEALS USED WAS TIME-SENSITIVE PLANNING WHERE WE PLANNED LITERALLY ON THE FLY AND COULD BE ON TARGET swifter than any other SOF unity. For our purposes here, with the strategy of mastering the breath, one tactic we will employ is box breathing, and another will be connecting breath with movement. Strategies without solid tactics lack punch. Tactics without an effective strategy don't get us through to mission accomplishment. We have ten core tactics that are employed to ensure our strategies put us on target.

TACTIC 1: SEQUENCING AND ADAPTATION

The sequencing in Kokoro Yoga refers to the order of poses in a given training session. By adeptly choosing and sequencing a series of poses for a purposeful session, along with variables such as how long you hold each individual pose and the breathing patterns used in the session, you can achieve different physical and mental results supporting your purposes. For example, a guiding purpose of the morning ritual is to stimulate your nervous system and enliven the spine so you are ready to move into your day alert, energized, and feeling powerful. Therefore, this practice includes poses, a sequence, and breathing patterns different from what you would perform in the evening ritual, where the intention is to move toward calmness and rest.

Part of my personal education in teaching yoga has included many hours in learning effective sequencing from a master, Gary Kraftsow. It's an art that's beyond the scope of this book, so we've created programming for a number of common-use scenarios, including the morning and evening practice, pre- and post-workout practice, stress management (Peaceful Warrior), functional fitness (Fit Warrior and Protective Warrior), warriorlike focus (Zen Warrior), and warrior energy development (Jedi Warrior).

Let's talk more about the principle of adaptation. I don't subscribe to the belief that the body must be contorted into some ideal pose. There's no demand being made that you have to funnel your body into the dream lotus position, or be able to execute a headstand that rewards you with a perfect 10 score. I have seen such a mind-set lead to frustration, injury, or both. Let us reverse that thinking. Rather than adapting your body to a pose, adapt the pose to what your body is ready for and capable of. I'd like you take into account who you are today and what you are dealing with as you approach your practice. Do you have old injuries that need to be considered? Most of us do. What about mobility restrictions? I'd be surprised if you don't have any. How does your age and experience impact your pose? All of these factors, and more, count. Please do not use this as an excuse to avoid riding the edge a bit, but know that it is fine not to be "perfect" and to leverage support tools, if necessary, like a folded blanket or a yoga block, to assist you into getting into a version of a pose that's right for you, at that moment.

TACTIC 2: CULTIVATING STILLNESS

There are several ways I want you to think about the tactic of cultivating stillness. At the physical level, let's picture you in the midst of performing a sequence of poses in your morning ritual. You will transition from pose to pose with a flowing style of movement. But in the full expression of the pose, we will take a few moments, measured with the breath, to practice stillness where we focus on being mindfully present. An example is when we hold the Downward-Facing Dog (aka Downward Dog or Down Dog) position for 8 or 10 breaths.

Another way to employ this tactic is the more advanced skill of finding stillness while moving. This is a place where we refrain from any mental and emotional distractions and sink our awareness into the movement itself. We aren't wondering about our ability to do the pose, or checking out the other students. Our mind is fully merged with the action; subject and object become one, experienced as embodied presence and stillness while moving. This deep internal awareness helps to unlock that flow state described earlier. A third way that we practice this tactic is in seated box breathing, visualization, and meditation drills. Even though our bodies are seemingly in a still position, there's still a lot of motion (i.e., our breathing patterns, fidgeting, and thinking of things you don't want or need to think about). During these sessions we want to pay attention to the motion in body, mind, and emotions, and strive to move toward stillness.

TACTIC 3: BREATH CONTROL

Breath control training will change your body and mind in remarkably positive ways. It will tune your nervous system and allow you to activate the parasympathetic or sympathetic nervous systems at will, helping you to perform in a stressful environment or to excel in competition. It will also place in your toolbox an immediate action drill to calm and focus your mind when necessary. Breath control training creates another "aha" moment for all of my students. It is so powerful and impacts you so quickly that you will wonder why such an important skill was kept from us our entire lives. I have selected some simple, yet profound, breathing practices to jump-start your training.

3-Part Breath

The first is to retrain the way we breathe from the ground up, or should I say the belly up. We will segment the breath into three parts to develop a new pattern of deep diaphragmatic breathing, one that utilizes our entire lung capacity. I call this the "3-Part Breath." To begin, place your hand on your belly, and take a deep inhalation through the nose. Picture your belly as if it were a balloon, and as you breathe in, inflate the belly balloon. Stop when your belly is fully extended, before you activate your diaphragm to deepen the breath even further.

Now when you exhale, blow all air out from the balloon through your nose while drawing the belly button back toward your spine; this will help you expunge all the remaining air. Repeat this first step 3 times. Okay, after 3 cycles, on the following inhalation, fill the belly up with air as in step one, but when the belly feels full, use your diaphragm to draw in more air, expanding the rib cage. Now when you expunge the breath, start with the air in the rib cage by allowing the ribs to compress back together, and then expel the remaining air from the belly. Repeat this second step a total of 3 times. The final stage of the 3-Part Breath is to once again fill the belly and activating the diaphragm to bring air into the rib cage, then you're going to top things off by expanding your rib cage and filling your chest all the way up to the collarbone with more air. Your upper chest will rise with expansion; the lungs will be completely full. You will note an energizing effect from the pressure. The sequence on the exhale will go from the top down: start by expelling the air from the upper chest, then the rib cage, then the belly. Notice the flow of relaxation that floods into your body on the exhale. Use this drill a couple times a day until you get the hang of breathing this way normally.

1:2 Breath

This breath control pattern is super simple and has the effect of calming you down and slowing your heart rate. This breathing technique uses a long, slow exhalation that triggers the parasympathetic, rest, and digest system into action. It counteracts your fight-or-flight system, which will calm down after just a few cycles. It is also a nice drill to begin to learn to control the duration of your inhale and exhale. It helps to practice this before you start to add holds such as with the box breathing drill.

The process is simply to exhale twice as long as you inhale. For instance, as you inhale through the nose using the full belly breath to a count of 3, you exhale out to a count of 6.

Over time, as your skill increases, you can take it to a 4:8 or 5:10 and so on. To yield some dramatic improvements with the 1:2 Breath, try a 30-day challenge of practicing it for 10 minutes each day. This is a great breathing pattern to use when in a stressful situation to gain control over your body and mind.

Box Breathing

The third breathing tactic will add a retention of the breath after inhale and exhale. This is my favorite breathing practice due to the powerful effect it has after only a short time of practicing. I gave it the name box breathing when I started doing it back in 2002 because of the four-sided pattern of the practice. It is something you can do anywhere and anytime you are not performing a highly complex task. I practice it in my morning ritual, before a workout, while standing in line, stuck in traffic, and whenever else I can. Along with training more powerful breathing musculature, it slows down the rate that you breathe and deepens your concentration skills. When you perform box breathing, even for 5 minutes, you are left with a deeply calm body and an alert, focused state of mind.

To begin the practice, expel all of the air from your chest. With empty lungs, retain this state for a 4-count hold. Press all the air out and then perform your inhalation, through the nose, to a count of 4. With the lungs full, hold for a count of 4. When you hold the breath, do not clamp down and create back pressure. Rather, maintain an expansive, open feeling even though you are not inhaling. When ready, release the hold and allow the exhale to flow out smoothly through your nose to a count of 4. This is one circuit of the box breathing practice. I recommend you do it for a minimum of 5 minutes, and no more than 20 minutes. I have found that the best approach is to do a single, dedicated practice of 10 to 20 minutes a day, then do a few 1- or 2-minute "spot drills" as opportunities present themselves during the day. Box breathing with this 4-4-4-4 ratio has a neutral energetic effect: It's not going to charge you up or put you into a sleepy relaxed state. But it will, as mentioned, make you very alert and grounded, ready for action. As your breathing threshold improves you can increase the duration of the ratio, such as 5-5-5-5 and so on.

Threshold Training

Would you like to increase the threshold of your lung capacity? Your breathing threshold is the duration of a complete breathing cycle, including any holds. It is determined by a few factors, such as the power of your breathing musculature, your lung capacity (volume of air they can hold), and the efficiency of gas transfer dictated by the strength of your heart's cardiac output (heart rate and stroke volume). If you have a threshold of 4 seconds then you are breathing 15 breaths per minute. Up to 20 cycles per minute is common, but don't read that as healthy. After years of practice, I now average 4 to 6 breaths per minute when not paying attention, and have a threshold of 55 seconds for a single breath, meaning I don't get winded or agitated with a 55 second breath count over a minimum of 12 cycles. The yoga masters believed that the human life span was determined by the number of breaths taken. According to them, slowing your breathing down would lengthen your life span. I don't know about you, but I am in—at 4 breaths per minute versus 16 I should live 4 times as long! At any rate, my experience is that slowing your breathing rate down is very healthy and I think you will find this to be true for yourself as well.

Let's begin threshold training with a ratio of 1:2:2:1. So a 3-second inhale, 6-second hold, 6-second exhale, and a 3-second hold is a 18-count breath threshold, assuming you can repeat this cycle comfortably a minimum of 12 times in a row. This would be just shy of three breaths per minute, which is a good target to work toward. For those who need to really extend your threshold, such as SEAL trainees, you will want to work toward a 60-second threshold. Note that you will be able to hold your breath longer in one-off situations when you prepare with sustained deep breathing and meditation. **Warning: never practice breath-hold training in the water alone.** I know it sounds obvious, but some special ops trainees have foolishly tried this and are not alive to read this book as a result.

TACTIC 4: FUNCTIONAL CONDITIONING

This tactic is one of the unique aspects of Kokoro Yoga—where we combine simple functional movements from SEALFIT training into an asana (pose) practice. This combination truly does turn the yoga session into an integrated workout. We should consider traditional yoga poses to be functional movements, (when done properly) but adding a module of interval exercises to your training session, such as with the Fit Warrior sequence, will build work capacity, strength, stamina, and durability. You may recall from chapter 1 that this is exactly what I did in Baghdad—adding 20-minute circuits of burpees, push-ups, jumping jacks, and Mountain Climbers in the middle of my yoga session. Another quick example: add a sequence of 20 sets of 5 push-ups, then 10 sets of 10 squats, and 5 sets of 20 sit-ups to break up your overall routine. In Appendix A, I share more sample functional workouts that you can use to employ this tactic. If this training inspires you and you have not been exposed to SEALFIT, I encourage you to check out my companion book, *8 Weeks to SEALFIT,* to learn a more challenging functional training regimen.

TACTIC 5: COMBAT CONDITIONING

This tactic brings yoga back to it's martial roots. I believe that a warrior must have a basic understanding of how to defend oneself. The foundation for self-defense is your mind, but it also requires the ability to make a weapon out of your body. Then you strike a desired target on another human being with those weapons if the need calls. Though Kokoro Yoga is not meant to be a martial art in the traditional sense, this tactic provides a fun and effective means to develop your punching and kicking weapons. You will get your heart rate up for a sustained period and break a good sweat, and you don't need a black belt to add this to your routine. If you can throw a punch and launch a kick, I hereby declare you ready to include the combat conditioning tactic to your practice.

A sample session would look like this: After a sequence of standing poses, you will insert 10 snap kicks with your right leg, then 10 left, followed by 10 punches with your right fist, and then 10 punches left. Next, you move on to some more complex combinations, or go back to your asana, then do it again a few more times during the training session. The possibilities are endless while being very empowering and fun. In Appendix B you will find more details on the movements and potential combinations.

TACTIC 6: AWARENESS AND RELAXATION

Awareness and relaxation work comes at the end of the session. With this tactic, your whole focus will turn inward with a full-body scan and breathing exercise that will prepare you for a meditation and visualization to mark the end of a session. The relaxation will help to integrate all of the benefits of the training session. As we do this, our internal sense of awareness deepens, leading to more sensitivity, composure, and depth. Recall the first strategy of developing a personal ethos? Well, deepening awareness is one way to gain insight into our deepest yearnings, leading to important growth…when we are ready.

This particular tactic is usually performed while in the Resting Pose (aka Dead Man Pose), though it can also be done in a seated meditation pose. With your eyes closed, you'll scan your body from toes to head, searching out pockets of tension, discomfort, and lingering emotions. The idea is not to judge these items but rather tune into each with neutral awareness. I should mention that this tactic is also a great place to work on your emotional development. As you scan you may notice emotions, and can take a few moments to explore the emotion in a detached way, examining the roots of the emotion. Now shift to a seated meditation position and move your awareness up your body, take time to pause at each of the six energy "cakra" centers:

ROOT: located at the base of your spine, associated with security and groundedness.

SACRAL: located about 3 inches above the root in your lower abdomen, below the navel, near the sacrum, associated with creativity.

BELLY: located just behind the belly button, associated with feelings of personal power.

HEART: located near the solar plexus and heart, associated with empathy and connecting to others.

THROAT: located in the throat region behind the Adam's apple, associated with sincere communication.

BROW: the third eye, so to speak, in the center head above cervical spine, associated with insight and wisdom.

CROWN: located at the top of the head, associated with universal connection and intelligence.

After this, take time to be aware of the surroundings and connect with the energy all around you.

TACTIC 7: CONCENTRATION AND MEDITATION

Concentration and meditation form another crucial tactic, and though they may sound one and the same, from the outside, there is a distinct difference in what is going on inside. Concentration is the skill of being able to maintain deep focus on one thing for long periods of time. It is one of the skills you are working on during your pose sequences and breathing exercises, where you are absorbed in a single, specific thing, rather than letting the mind run. As mentioned, daily asana and box breathing drills are tremendous at improving your concentration. When you are concentrating, you are deeply engaged in observing the object of attention, so that you can maintain that focus for long periods of time without distraction. Concentrating with this depth is particularly useful for creative work, reading, problem-solving, or observing a target. In concentration your eyes will be focused intently, and your center of consciousness is in your critical thinking mind. Even if just practicing box breathing, you are focused intently on the breathing pattern, the quality of the breath, and the experience itself.

Meditation differs in that you will observe an object, a mantra, or some concept with complete absorption and presence, not using your critical thinking mind, rather allowing for direct perception to occur. Ultimately you will sense a merging with the object of your attention. This is a good place to mention that your mind works in five distinct ways: critical thinking (judging, analyzing, deciding), direct perception (just observing and knowing things without judging), imagining things, accessing memory, and dreaming. Interestingly, the way you use your eyes and the region of your brain that is active differs with each mode. When you meditate your eyes will be closed, or if open they will be soft, wide, and not focused. When you concentrate your eyes are piercing, focused.

The practice of meditation is difficult but, ironically, practicing a form of concentration first makes it easier. That is because training your mind in concentration allows us to collapse the myriad of thoughts to just one or two and helps us to still the active mind. When we begin to meditate we are less distracted. Within a few months of consistent concentration practice, you will note that you are more present. Your mind has developed resistance to being swept away with worries and distractions. You will begin to identify with the witnessing part of you, rather than with the thoughts themselves.

Not all meditation is focused on an object, mantra, or concept. In mindful meditation, an adaptation of a Buddhist meditative practice, we seek a state of non-judging awareness where sensory input, such as a car honking its horn or a thought of an important task, is noticed without judgment, attachment, and upending our equanimity. We just notice the disturbance and instantly let it go. As we get into higher and higher stages of meditation, we are able to shut down the noise of the mind entirely and rest in a deeply absorbed state. At that level of progress you will begin to experience shibumi, which was described in the last chapter. You will want to experiment with objects of concentration and forms of meditation to determine what is best for your personality and stage of development. Seeking guidance from an expert is very helpful with this tactic.

TACTIC 8: VISUALIZATION

I have relied on visualization practice since I used it to both get into and through the rigorous SEAL training back in 1990. With Kokoro Yoga we strive to train the brain's ability to create and hold imagery so that we can imagine, then see with clarity, something we desire to achieve in the future, or to learn from in the past. This tactic specifically works on your mental and wisdom dimensions. With visualization we can create imagery for an intended purpose, and repeatedly revisit said imagery to develop a skill, heal, gain insights on something, or to develop confidence and momentum toward completing a goal. A familiar and powerful use of visualization training is to prepare for a competition by visualizing your best performance, whether real or imagined. This practice will cut a mental, emotional, and nervous system groove upon which to follow as you perform. Research has proven that most skills can be improved through visualization. For example, imagining perfect technique in successful free throw basketball shots, we can markedly enhance the development of that skill.

I'd like to emphasize some of the more important uses for visualization work. As alluded to, I first employed this tactic when I was preparing for Basic Underwater Demolition SEAL training. For 9 months I spent time daily visualizing myself as a Navy SEAL, as having successfully completed the program, and wearing the SEAL Trident. The visualization slowly rendered within me an overwhelming level of belief that I was destined to be a SEAL. By the time I arrived in Coronado to begin the training, I had already won in my mind. The training was familiar and I had a deep sense of confidence that I would succeed. Nothing could get in my way, and I credit the visualization training for reinforcing my mental toughness and resiliency. Visualization practice can sow seeds deep within to help you achieve goals, develop healthy self-esteem, and untangle psychological blocks. I have also seen its effectiveness in treating PTSD and emotional abuse. There are several visualization exercises described in chapter 6 to get you started. This tactic is typically employed at the close of a training session, but can also be done as a stand-alone drill.

TACTIC 9: SPOT DRILLS

Kokoro Yoga is designed for busy individuals who may at first wonder how they're going to jam yet another activity into their already overwrought schedules. This ninth tactic will allow you to integrate several drills into a single ritual or workout, and to do your training "on the spot" in the many free spots that open up during the day. This tactic also comes from my original experience in Baghdad. Time was extremely limited—I had to skip breakfast for training in the first place. But during the long days and nights, I would still get physically fatigued, mentally cluttered, or emotionally charged. So I relied on spot drills to get back into balance and maintain a link with my integrated training. Bottom line, if you can breathe, then you can train! Most of the drills take just 1 or 2 minutes, and even on the most hectic days you can be innovative and locate a few minutes here or there that might otherwise go wasted. Waiting in line, browsing the net, driving your car, visiting the restroom, on board an airplane—if you aren't engaged in a conversation, you can be doing a 1-minute (or longer) movement, breathing, concentration, memory, mental agility, or visualization practice. When flying, there's no harm in going to the back of the cabin and figuring out a pose or two that you can do. At the office, set your alarm so that on the hour, you take a minute to do a Sun Salutation or box breathing. Develop the habit of choosing 2 in the morning and 2 in the afternoon. Here are a few ideas to get you started:

- Short breathing drill

- Sun Salutation A

- 1 minute of mindful awareness meditation

- 1-minute body scan

- What wolf are you feeding? check-in. Ask if you are in a positive frame of mind or stuck in the negative. If positive, reinforce it. If negative, interdict and redirect to positive.

- Recite a powerful mantra or affirmation. My favorite: "Feeling good, looking good, oughta be in Hollywood."

- Listen to an empowering podcast.

- Read a poem, bible verse, or a paragraph in an inspiring book.

- Visualize the alphabet in large, neon letters, drawing each letter mentally.

- Use a brain-training app for mental speed, agility, and improving memory.

- Ask what you are grateful for.

- Chant.

- Express gratitude to a coworker, spouse, child, or boss.

- Smile for a full minute.

- Laugh out loud for a while—laughing yoga is a powerful positive boost and a blast!

Spot drilling is a habit that you can weave into your life. After all, life is just a big training ground. Over time, these spot drills will accelerate and compound your training, making a profound difference in your life.

TACTIC 10: AUSTERE AND TRAVEL TRAINING

I've included this tactic because I want you to realize, first of all, you don't need spandex pants, a yoga studio, or $300 of equipment to practice Kokoro Yoga. And second—as indicated in the previous tactic—no matter how busy you are or how much you travel, the original nature of yoga was to be versatile so that you can make any location suitable for a great training session. If you have 5 minutes to an hour, and access to any open space, you are good to go. As far as yoga studios, getting outside has myriad perks. A nature trail is a wonderful place to do your practice. I personally love to step away from the gym and go down to the beach to train among the waves and seagulls. When traveling, the airport concourse and the patch of free space in front of my hotel bed are my studios.

As far as equipment, you really don't need much—even a yoga mat is a luxury sometimes. Ninety-nine percent of what you need is carried on your body and between your ears. Straps, blocks, or towels are easy to come by and a meditation bench is easy to make. For functional fitness equipment I encourage you to scrounge through your garage or basement to find things to pick up and move that will serve you well. If you want to buy the gear go ahead, but it can also be fun to employ the austerity measure of this tactic and improvise to overcome. If austere training is new, it may surprise you to learn just how fun and challenging training with a bag of sand can be!

Bottom line: This training allows for no excuses. Now let's learn the classic poses and get moving.

CHAPTER 5

CORE
SEQUENCES

Watching [Norman] do his practice was like watching an Olympic gymnast work out.

—BERYL BENDER BIRCH, DESCRIBING HIS FIRST IMPRESSIONS OF ASHTANGA YOGA IN 1955

KOKORO YOGA HAS STEADILY EVOLVED OVER THE YEARS SINCE ITS INCEPTION IN THE CARGO HOLD OF MY C-130 FLIGHT TO A WAR ZONE. THROUGH THIS DEVELOPMENT PERIOD I HAVE CONTINUED TO EDUCATE MYSELF IN THE PHILOSOPHY AND THE PRACTICE OF THE ANCIENT ARTS AND DEVELOPED PROGRAMS TO ASSIST OTHERS IN LEARNING. MY DRIVE HAS BEEN TO INSPIRE OTHERS TO LIVE BY A PERSONAL ETHOS AND DEVELOP A DISCIPLINED TRAINING IN THE FIVE MOUNTAINS—

both of which are anchored in the ancient yoga traditions as well as elite modern warrior training. Personal development of this nature closes the openings of our weaknesses and leverages our strengths, ultimately balancing physical, mental, emotional, intuitional, and spiritual aspects of our lives. This chapter will delve into the actual training routines called sequences. Here you will learn the core sequences to employ in your daily lives as you develop your own training plan and personal practice.

TRAINING AND PRACTICE

To experience the full benefits of a practice, one must select a training regimen with appropriate tools, and practice daily, weekly, and monthly. Often the training is just referred to as "practice" —Ashtanga Yoga founder Sri K. Pattabhi Jois reminds us that: "Yoga is 99% practice, 1% theory" and "practice, and all else is coming!" The effective employment of yoga requires that we understand and properly employ the training methods, as well as develop a personal practice suitable to our lives. Training methods will be discussed in this chapter, and developing a personal practice will be the focus of chapter 8.

Training and practice are definitely related and are often used synonymously, but they are different concepts. As mentioned, training refers to a regimen, a method, and also an event, such as a training session or seminar. Training covers strategies, tactics, and tools available for practitioners of the system of development. It is highly unlikely that a practitioner will use all of the strategies, tactics, and tools available. Rather, he or she will select the appropriate ones for them and construct a training regimen to meet their specific objectives. This is where training begins to overlap with the concept of a personal practice. Even though two people may be using the same tools and similar training regimen, they will each approach it in an individualized manner of personal practice. Rather than just pulling a sequence or drill out of a box and doing it for a training session, you will select those most appropriate for your life situation and weave them into a daily, weekly, and monthly practice that supports and improves your lifestyle. That is why it is called a personal practice—it is deeply personal to you and no two personal practices are the same.

At any rate, in deciding how to construct your training plan you will begin with your intentional needs (which will change over time), your fitness level (which will also evolve), and your work/life situation. So rather than just showing up randomly at a yoga studio and getting your sweat on, you ask yourself: What is my intention with the practice overall and for this particular period of my life. This includes what warrior archetype you seek to develop further. For example, my stepdaughter Catherine, who leads our teacher training program and has coauthored this book, answers this question with: "I am a warrior of peace, and it is my intention to spread love into the world through my teaching and personal practice." Catherine's deep experience teaching and practicing yoga and meditation brings a gentle side to her warrior archetype. She organizes her training to support that archetype and development. It includes a selection of gentle and restorative sequences, meditation, and Ashtanga and Viniyoga skills.

My training plan differs because as a retired SEAL and teacher of warriors, I strive to remain grounded in the combat warrior way as well as develop my kokoro spirit. I need to be a protector and ready for battle at all times. I strive to ride my razor's edge so I can always lead by example. I do this to stay true to my stand and align with my purpose of mastering myself so I can serve and inspire others. My principles include earning my trident of respect every day, so I endeavor for daily improvement. All of this is in search of continuous, conscious evolution that will help me authentically serve others in their own journey. To support my training I do the morning and evening rituals every day, as well as teach or perform the more rigorous Protective Warrior and Fit Warrior sequences once or twice a week. I also train with box breathing, meditation, my mantra, and visualization once or more times a day. We will look at how Catherine and I organize these training methods into our personal practice in chapter 8.

SEQUENCING

Sequences are one of the primary tools of an effective yoga system. Sequences combine poses, breathing methods, functional fitness, combat conditioning moves, visualization and meditation into focused and intentional training regimens. Recall that sequencing the movements into an intelligent flow, that fulfills a distinct purpose, is the first strategy of Kokoro Yoga. Learning to sequence effectively takes many years of experience, so we have designed sequences for you that meet the most common applications of a personal practice. One sequence will challenge the elite warrior, another will appeal to the peaceful warrior and yet another will support the warrior in need of psychological and spiritual recovery. Applying the right sequence at the right moments in your training plan, and in life, is potent medicine.

What follows are select sequences to get you started on your journey. Please explore them with the intuitive sense of your needs and let experience be your guide. It is a good idea to review the pose descriptions and pictures in chapter 7 before trying out these sequences.

The Core Sequences

The core sequences are practice sessions of varying length that meet specific training objectives. Your objectives will vary, but we wanted to cover a few that every healthy practitioner can benefit from.

I am particularly excited to offer a sequence for warriors recovering from intense stress or career-related psychological wounds. I have no doubt about the value of this sequence in assisting wounded warriors to recover and find balance and peace again.

The sequences are included in written form at the end of this chapter, but it is awkward to describe the sequences themselves with words. Therefore we have included photos (with accompanying captions) to help visually demonstrate the pose/sequence.

In each of the core sequences the poses are linked with the breath. Additionally some poses are held for a set number of breaths (indicated in the written version). One of the distinctions of Kokoro Yoga is the adaptable nature of the poses, so that even a beginner can do any of the sequences by modifying: Some pose modifications are shown.

Peaceful Warrior

The Peaceful Warrior is approximately 45 minutes long and will take you deep into an inner state of peace and leave you feeling very grounded. It will provide a moderate level of endurance training and has a broad focus on spinal and joint health as well as energetic alignment. Bring your Peaceful Warrior attitude to this practice.

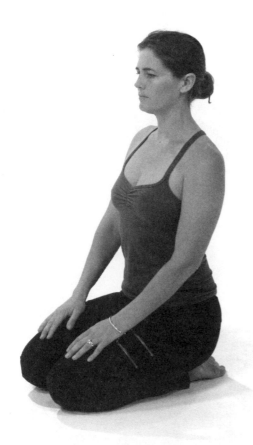

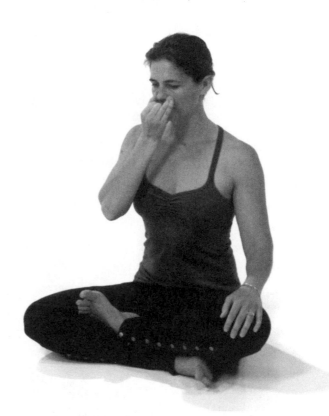

SEATED MEDITATION— SET INTENTION
PW1

ALTERNATE NOSTRIL BREATHING
PW2

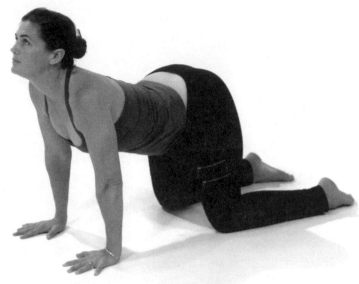

PW3

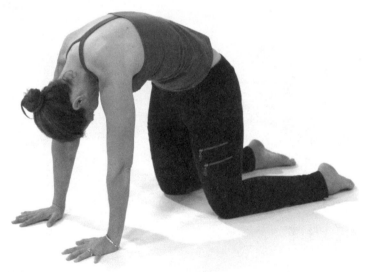

PW4

CAT COW ROTATION

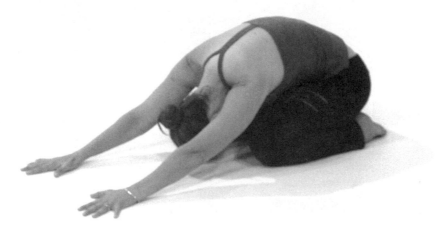

PW5

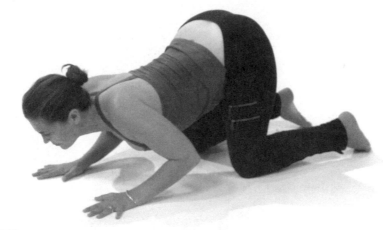

PW6

DOWNWARD DOG

**TRANSITION BACK
TO DOWN DOG**
PW7

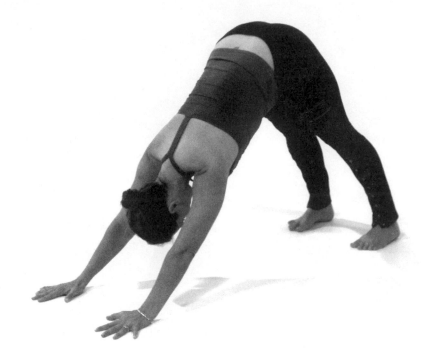

KNEELING WARRIOR—
EACH SIDE

PW8

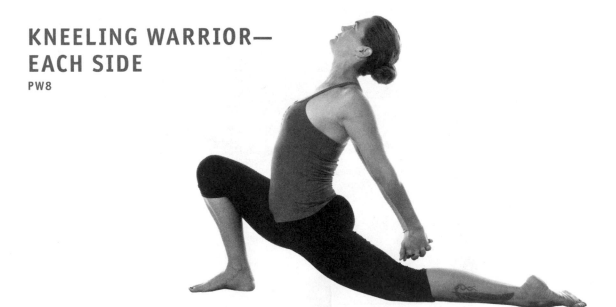

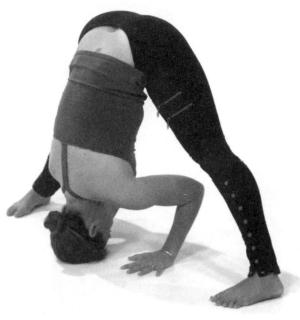

WIDE ANGLE
FORWARD FOLD
PW9

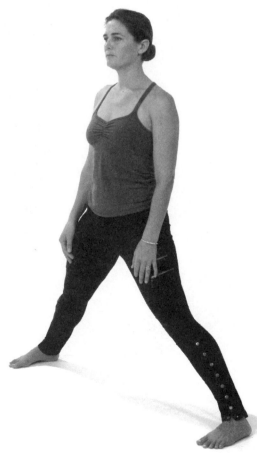

ROLL UP TO
STANDING
PW10

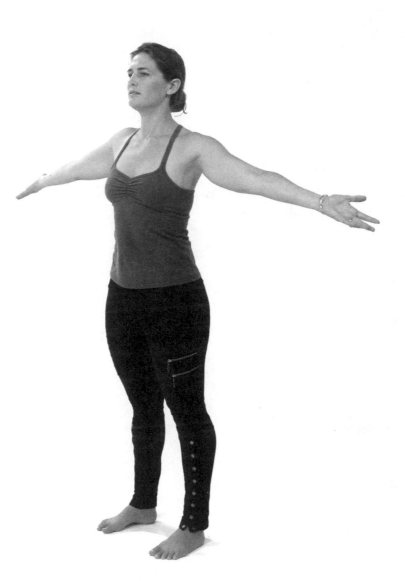
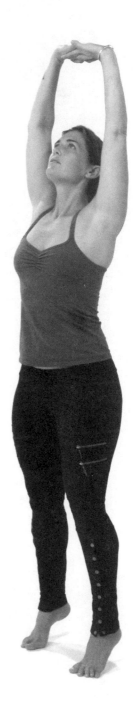

BRINGING DOWN THE HEAVENS 3X
PW11A

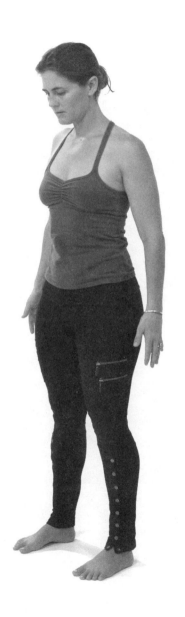

SUN SAL AX2

SUN SALUTATION A—2X

PW11B

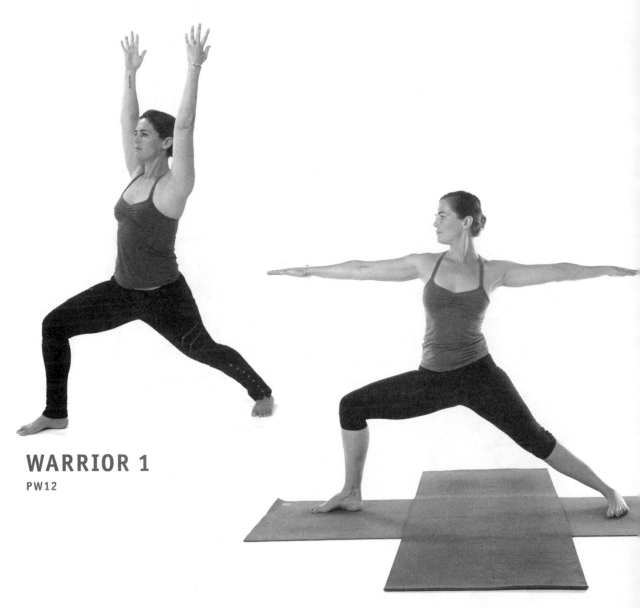

WARRIOR 1

PW12

WARRIOR 2

PW13

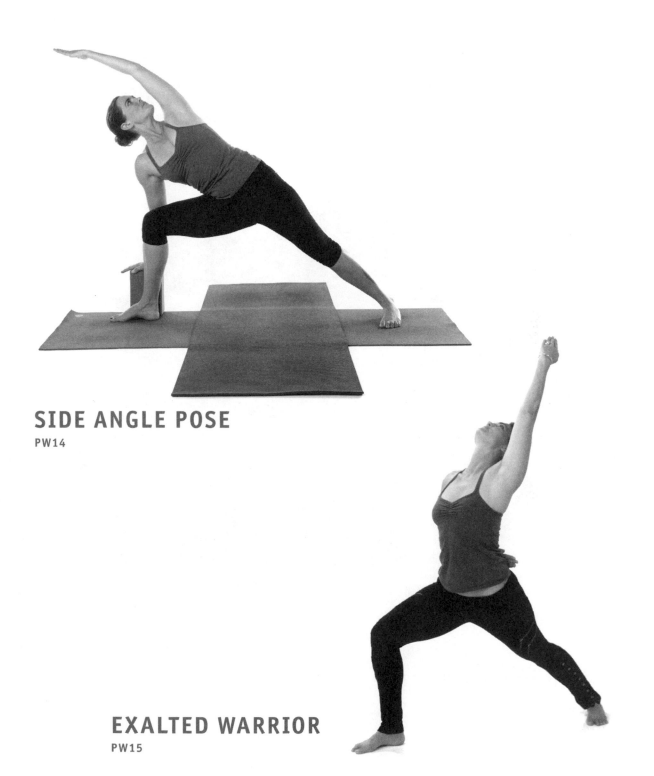

SIDE ANGLE POSE
PW14

EXALTED WARRIOR
PW15

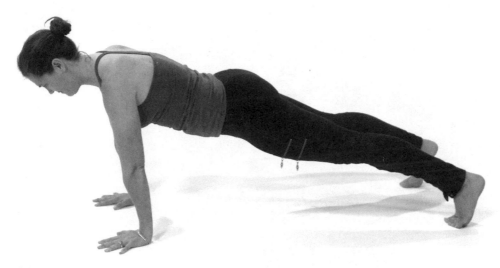

PW16

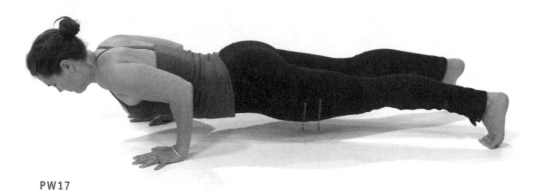

PW17

PUSH-UP PLANK

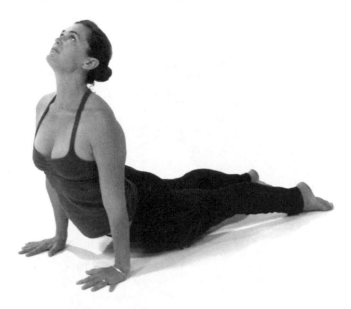

UPWARD-FACING DOG
PW18

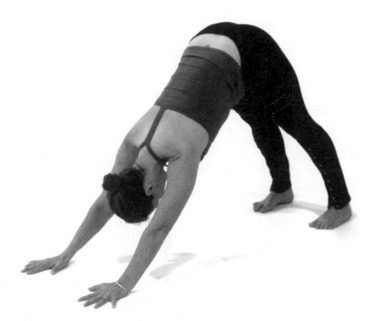

DOWNWARD DOG
REPEAT LEFT SIDE
PW19

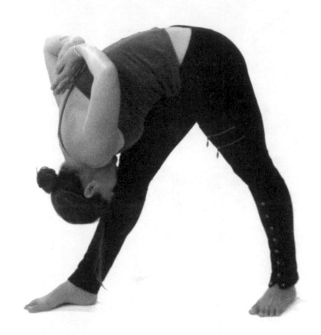

SHARP WARRIOR
PW20

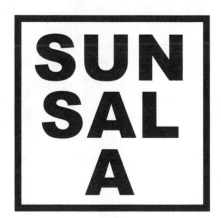

SUN SALUTATION A
PW21

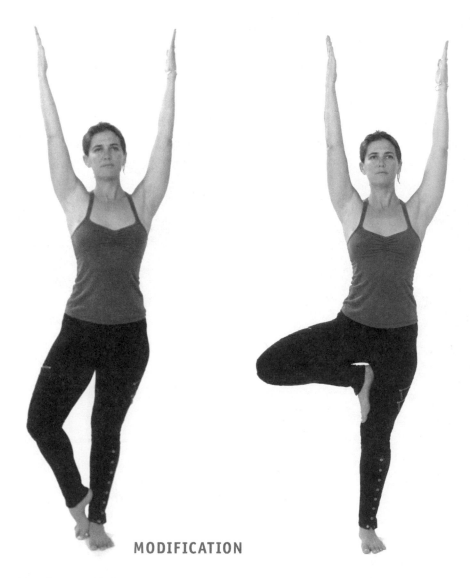

MODIFICATION

TREE POSE
PW22

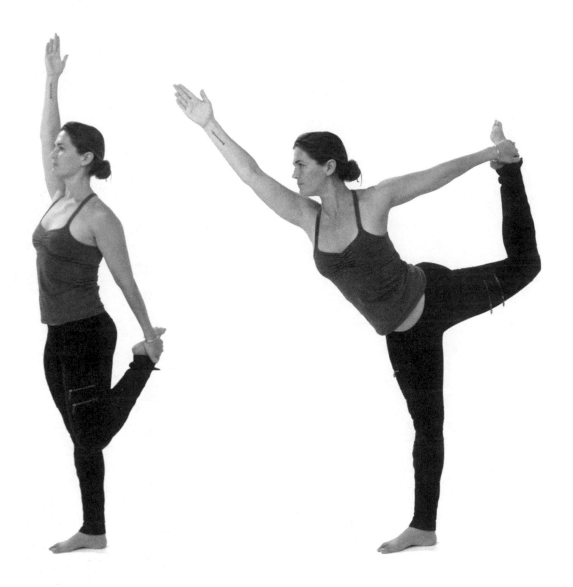

DANCER POSE

PW23

SUN SAL A

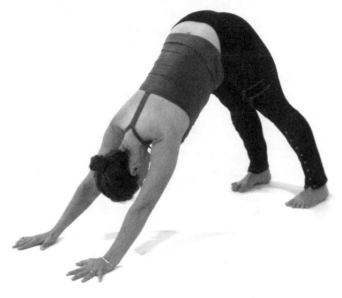

SUN SALUTATION A
TO DOWNWARD DOG—
THEN COME TO A SEAT
PW24

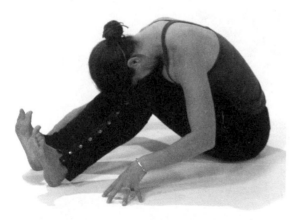

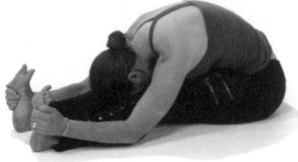

SEATED FORWARD FOLD
PW25

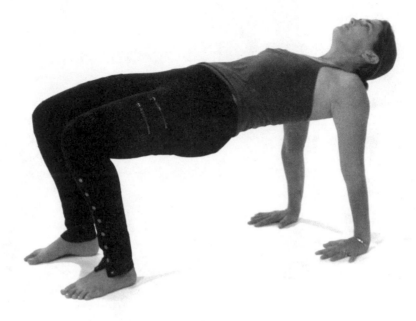

TABLETOP
PW26

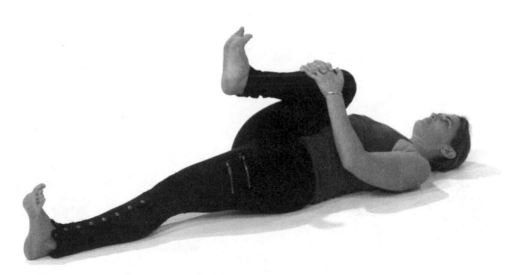

CLEANSING WARRIOR (EACH SIDE)
PW27

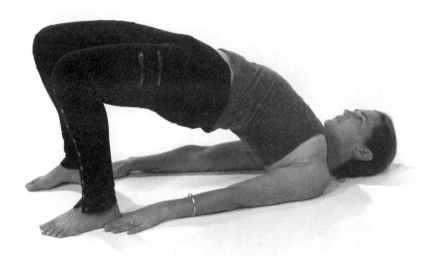

PW28

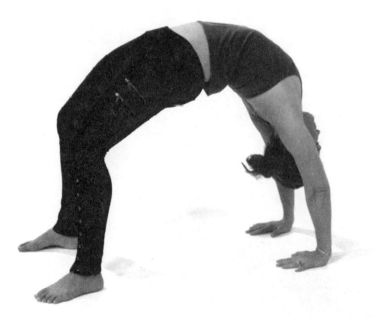

PW29

BRIDGE OR WHEEL—2X

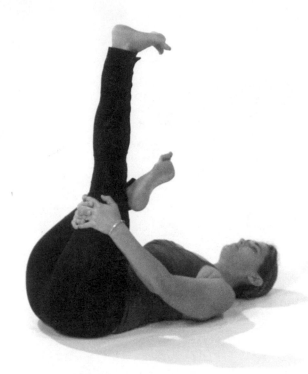

RECLINED PIGEON (EACH SIDE)
PW30

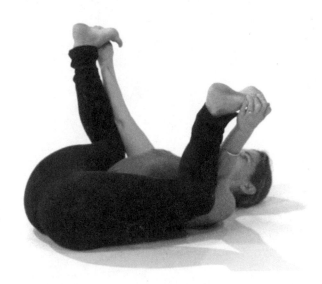

HAPPY BABY POSE
PW31

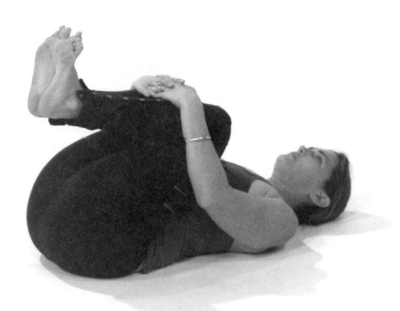

HEALTHY WARRIOR
PW32

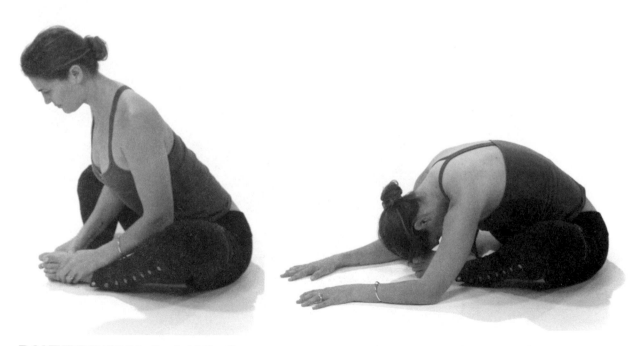

BUTTERFLY 1 AND 2
PW33

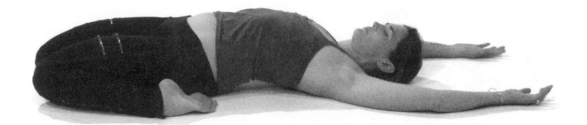

RECLINED WARRIOR POSE
PW34

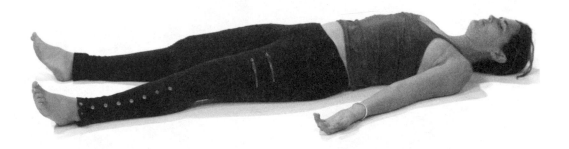

RESTING POSE
PW35

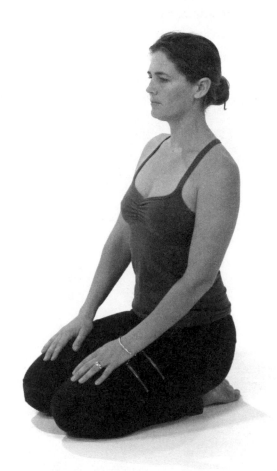

SEATED MEDITATION—
REVISIT INTENTION AND BREATH

COMPASSION AND PEACE MEDITATION
PW36

Zen Warrior

The Zen Warrior is a moderately challenging 30-minute long sequence. It will cultivate strength, flexibility, and enhance your ability to access a moving meditative state. It covers the standing warrior poses and breathing exercises, as well as some nice core development, backbends, and spinal twists. Most importantly, bring your serene and victorious warrior attitude into this practice. Use the time to sharpen your mental sword and find victory in your mind, like the samurai on the Zen bench prior to battle. Breath awareness is a key to maintain throughout the practice, as it will help awaken the flow state.

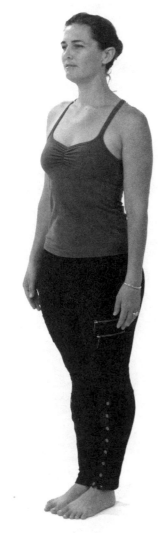

MOUNTAIN POSE

(5X 1–2 BREATHS)

ZW1

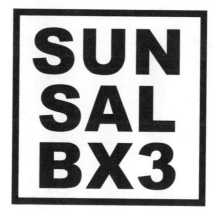

SUN SALUTATION A—3X

ZW2

SUN SALUTATION B—3X

ZW3

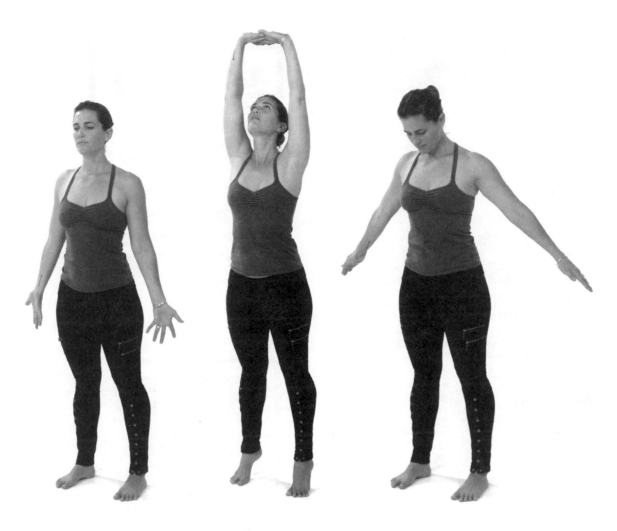

BRINGING DOWN THE HEAVENS

ZW4

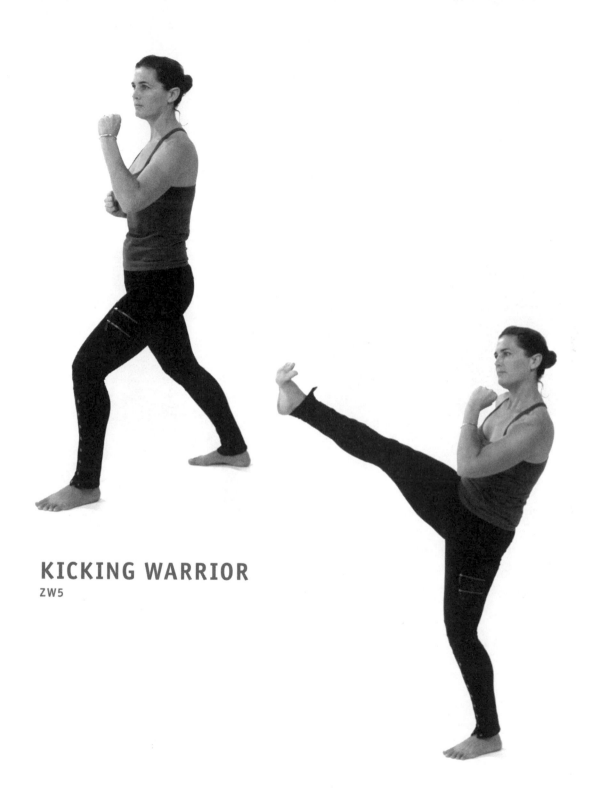

KICKING WARRIOR
ZW5

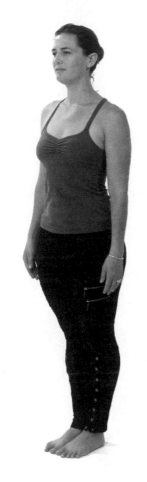

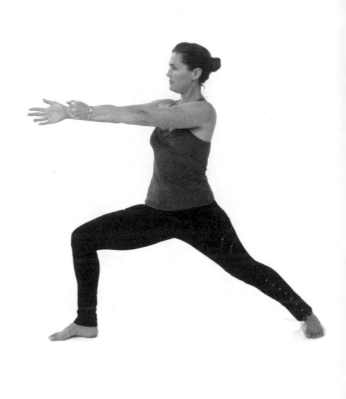

MOUNTAIN POSE

ZW6

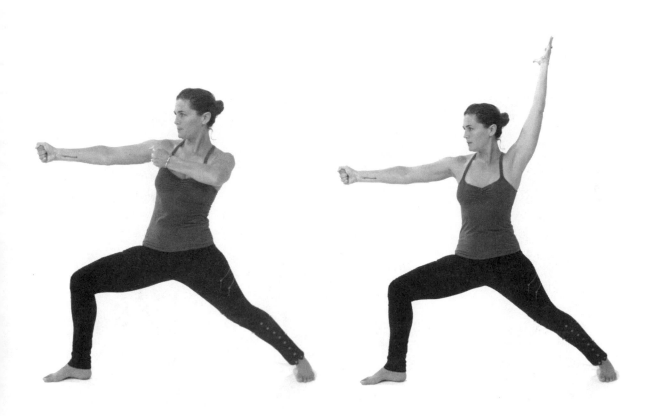

ARCHER WARRIOR

ZW7

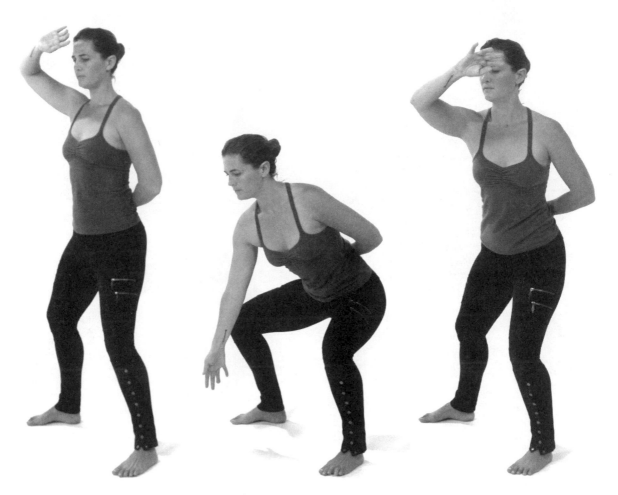

SCOOPING THE MOON
ZW8

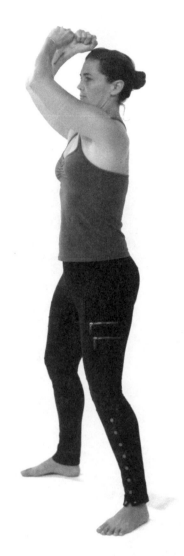
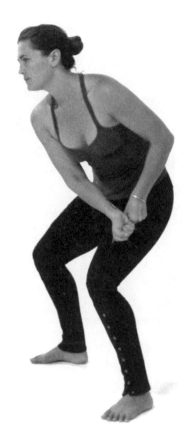

WARRIOR MUSASHI

ZW9

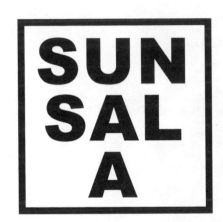

SUN SALUTATION A

Z10

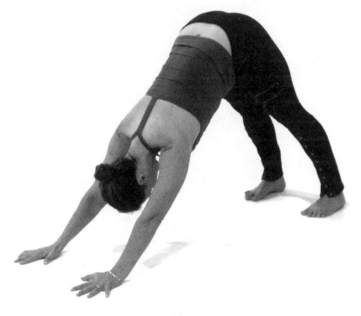

**DOWNWARD DOG—
COME TO KNEES**

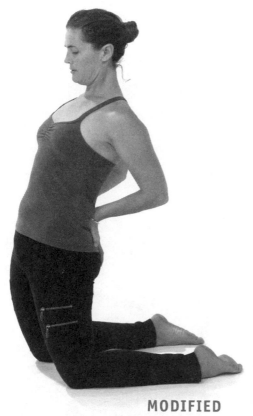

MODIFIED

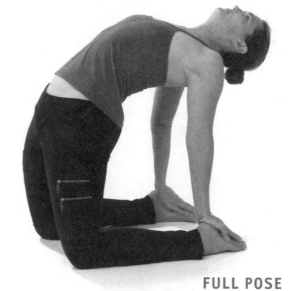

FULL POSE

CAMEL
Z11

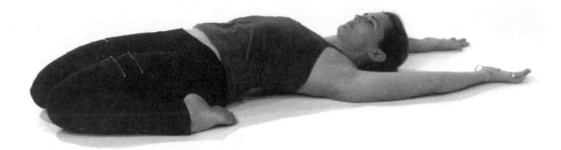

RECLINED WARRIOR POSE
ZW12

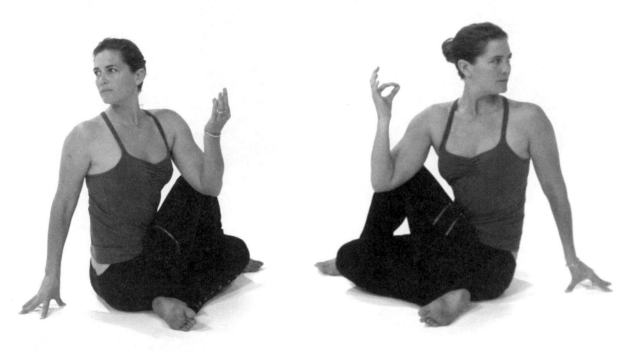

WISE WARRIOR TWIST
ZW13

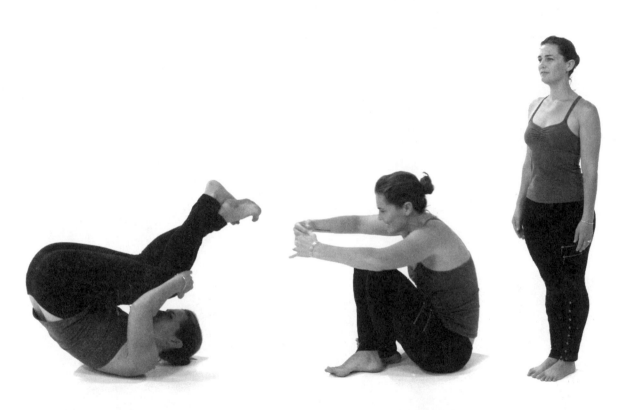

ROCK BACK AND FORTH TO STANDING
ZW14

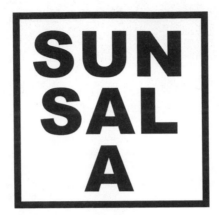

ZW15

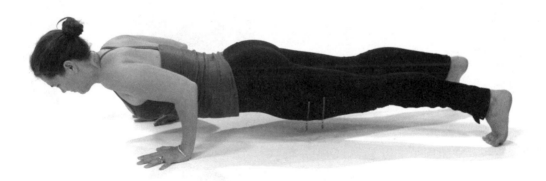

SUN SALUTATION A TO PUSH-UP— LOWER ONTO BELLY

ZW15

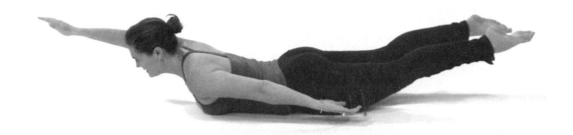

1-ARM LOCUST—EACH SIDE
ZW16

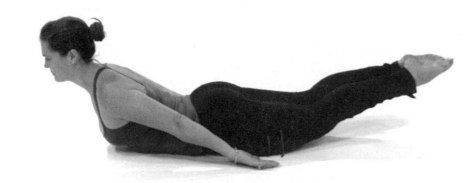

LOCUST
ZW17

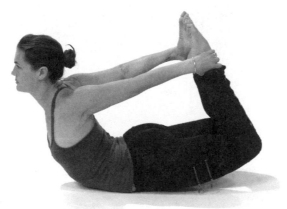

BOW
ZW18

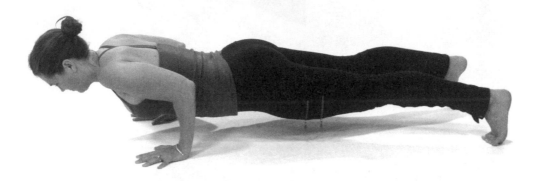

REVERSE PUSH-UP
ZW19

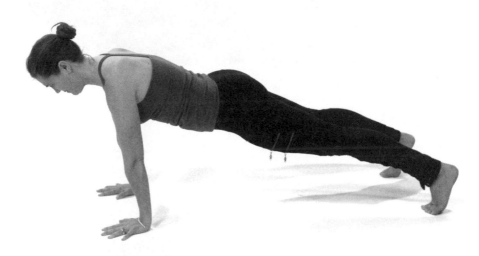

PUSH-UP—5X
ZW20

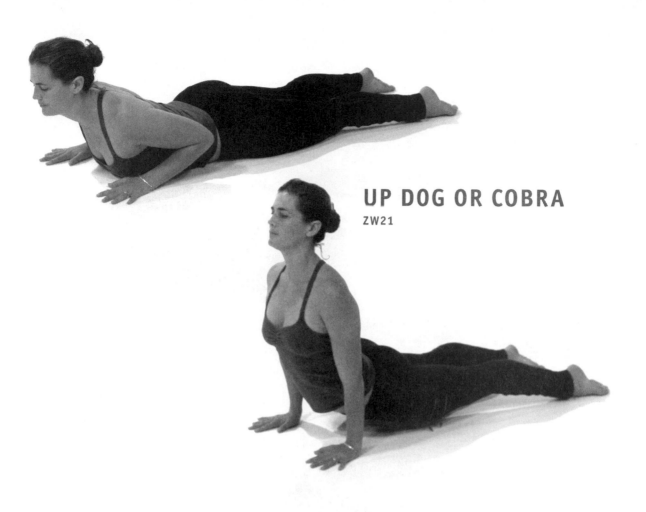

UP DOG OR COBRA
ZW21

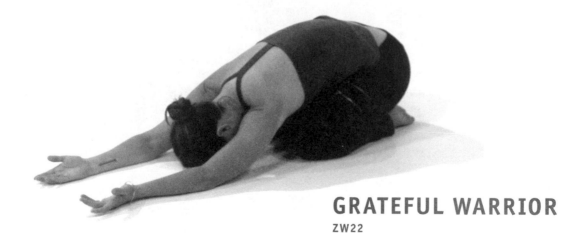

GRATEFUL WARRIOR
ZW22

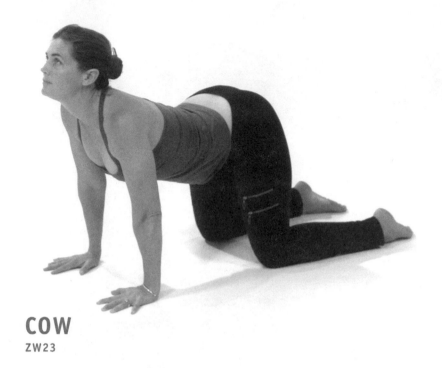

COW
ZW23

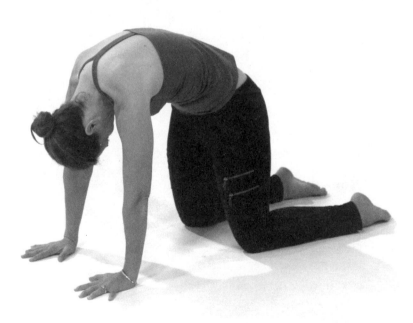

CAT
ZW24

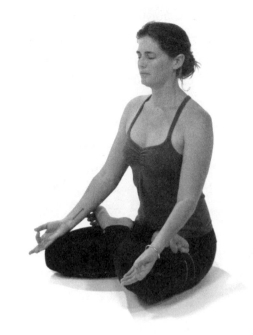

BOX
BREATHING
3-6-6-3 5X

ZW25

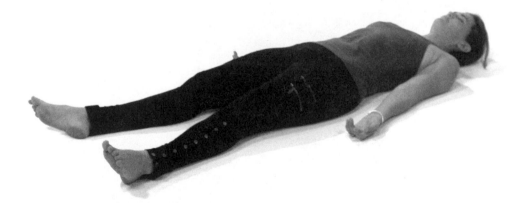

RESTING POSE

FOLLOW WITH STRENGTH AND GROUNDING MEDITATION

ZW26

Fit Warrior

The length of this sequence depends upon how long you do the functional fitness module. It is typically about a 45-minute dynamic flow with an intense interval-training component. It is definitely on the challenging end of the spectrum but can be scaled according to your needs. The session will take you deep inside your mental training space, while providing a kick-ass, fun workout to supplement your functional fitness training. This is a great sequence to use if you are a road warrior with limited access to weights and other tools; it is excellent for women who don't want to "throw weights around"; and for beginners or older trainees who are uncomfortable with weighted training. This sequence can be performed in two ways. This first is where the fitness segments are inserted into the middle as a distinct module. The second is to add the fitness movements throughout the sequence between the yoga poses, such as doing 10 push-ups after every other Up Dog, or 20 squats between the transition from one side to the other on warrior poses. Appendix B has a number of exercise combinations to choose from, or you can let your intuition guide you!

BOX
BREATHING
3-6-6-3 5X

FW1

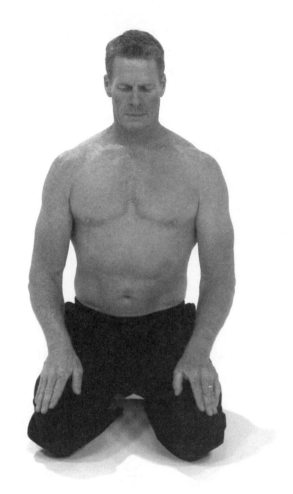

FW2

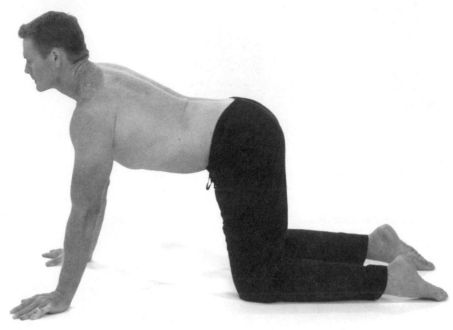

COW

FW3

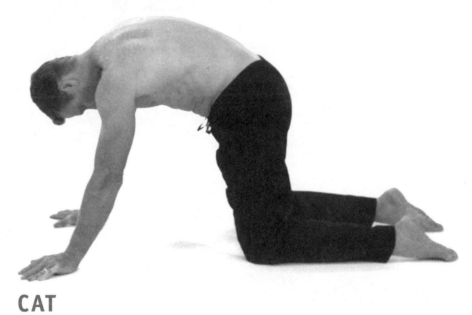

CAT

FW3

REPEAT OTHER SIDE

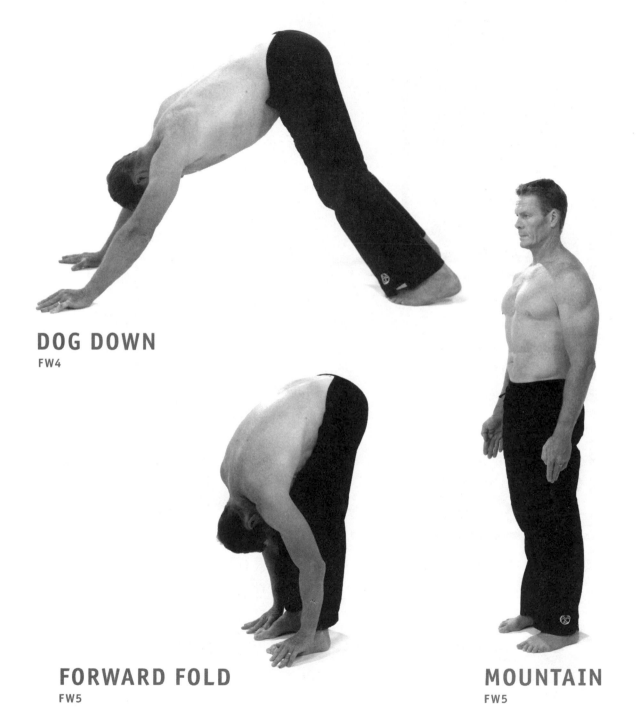

DOG DOWN
FW4

FORWARD FOLD
FW5

MOUNTAIN
FW5

SUN SAL AX2

SUN SALUTATION AX2
FW6

SUN SAL BX2

SUN SALUTATION AX2
FW7

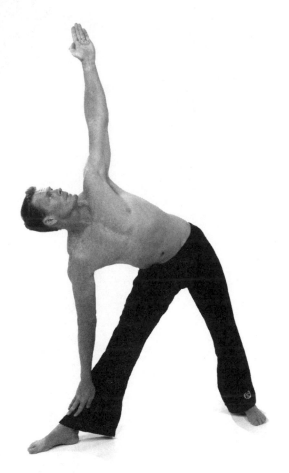

TRIANGLE
FW8

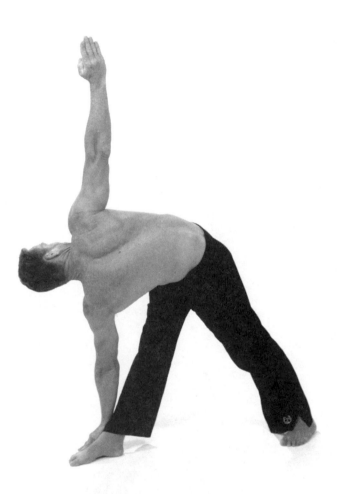

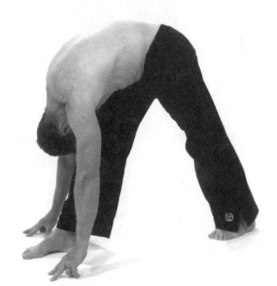

TWISTED TRIANGLE
FW9

SHARP WARRIOR
FW10

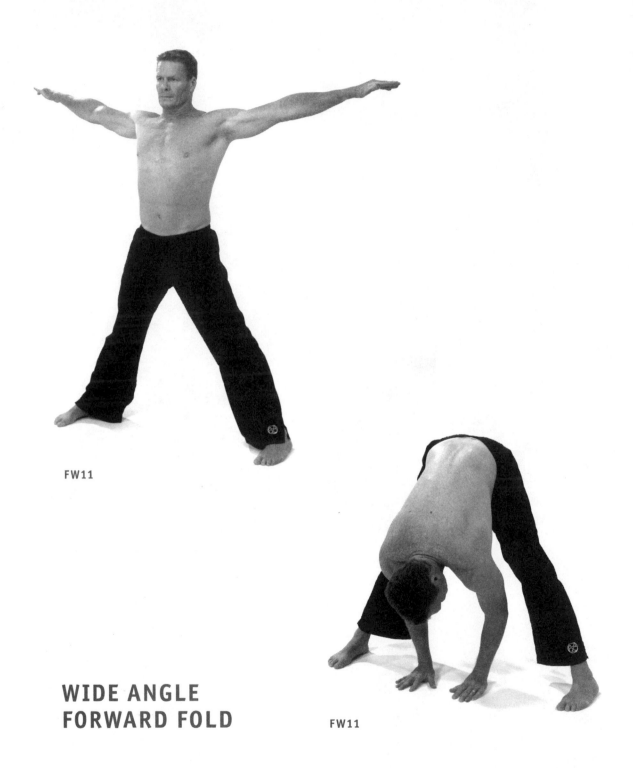

FW11

WIDE ANGLE FORWARD FOLD

FW11

Mark Divine and Catherine Divine

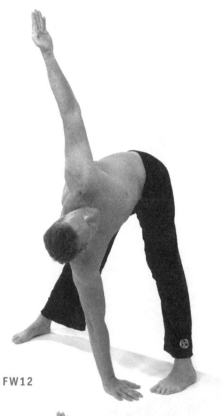

FW12

TWISTED WIDE ANGLE FORWARD FOLD

FW12

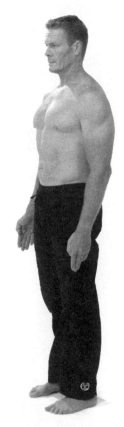

MOUNTAIN—REPEAT SEQUENCE ON LEFT SIDE

FW12

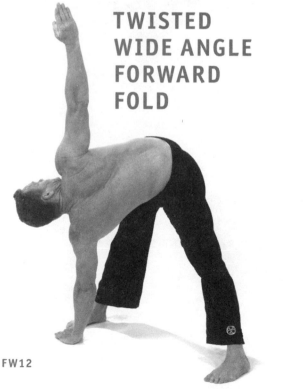

FW12

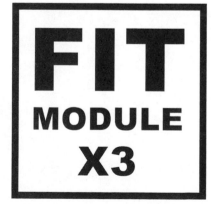

FIT MODULE X3

FW13

Fit Module

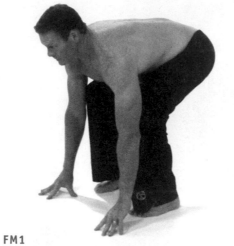

FM1

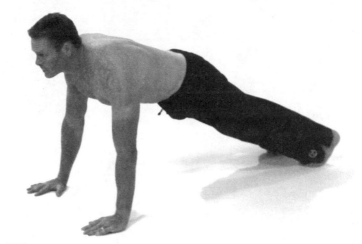

FM2

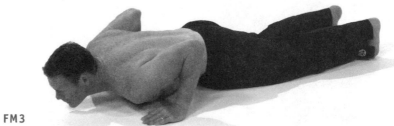

FM3

10 BURPEES

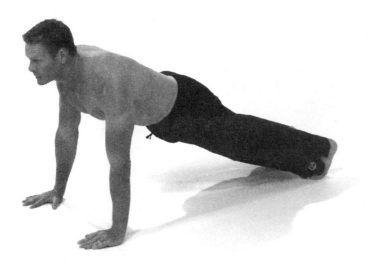

FM4

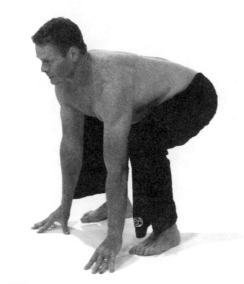

FM5

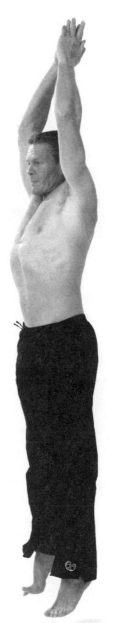

FM6

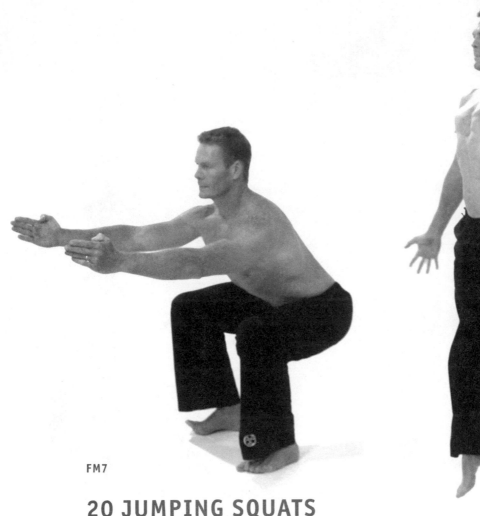

FM7

20 JUMPING SQUATS

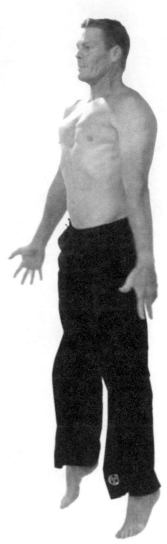

FM8

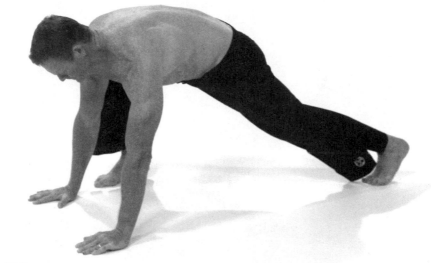

FM9

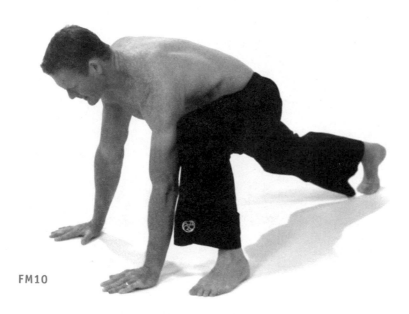

FM10

20 MOUNTAIN CLIMBERS

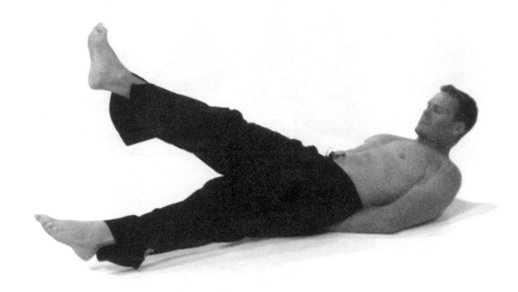

FM11

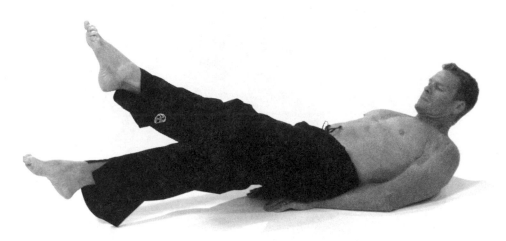

FM12

FLUTTER KICKS

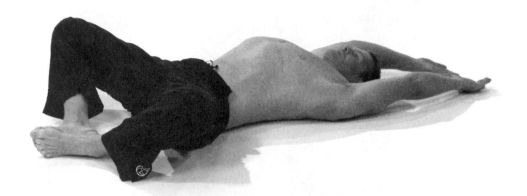

FM13

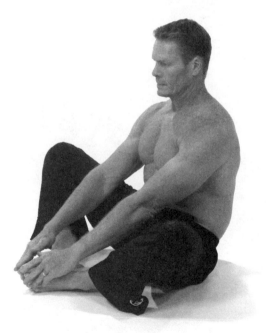

FM14

20 SIT-UPS

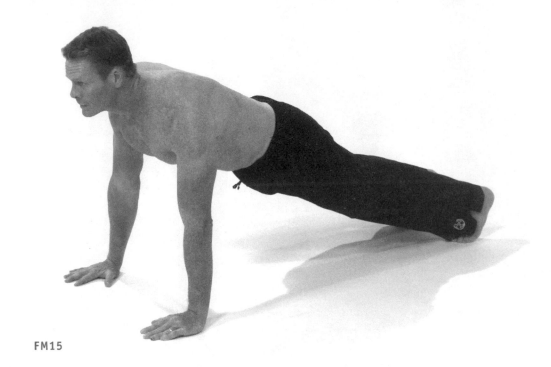

FM15

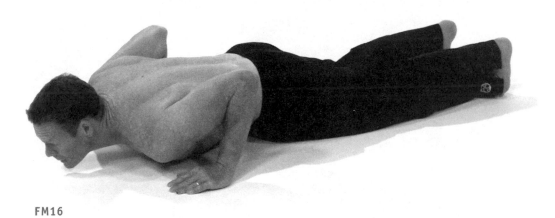

FM16

20 PUSH-UPS

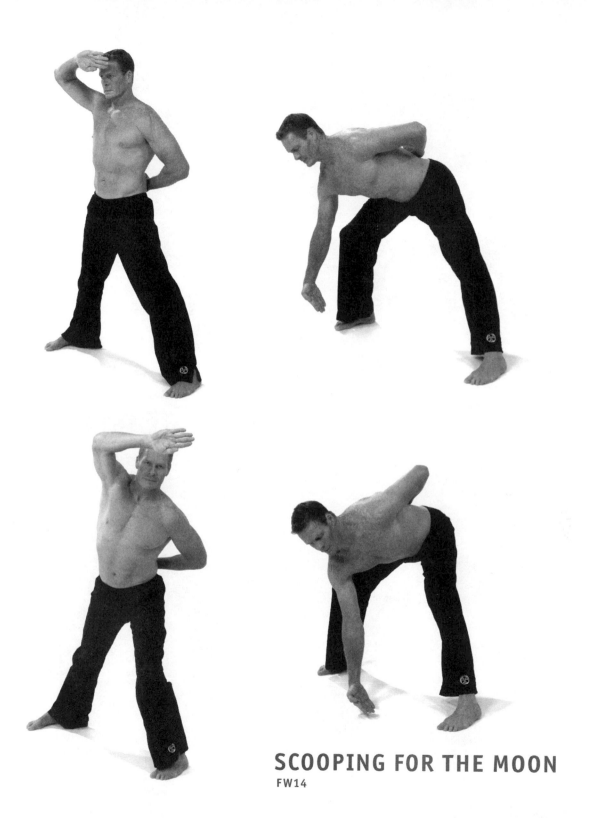

SCOOPING FOR THE MOON
FW14

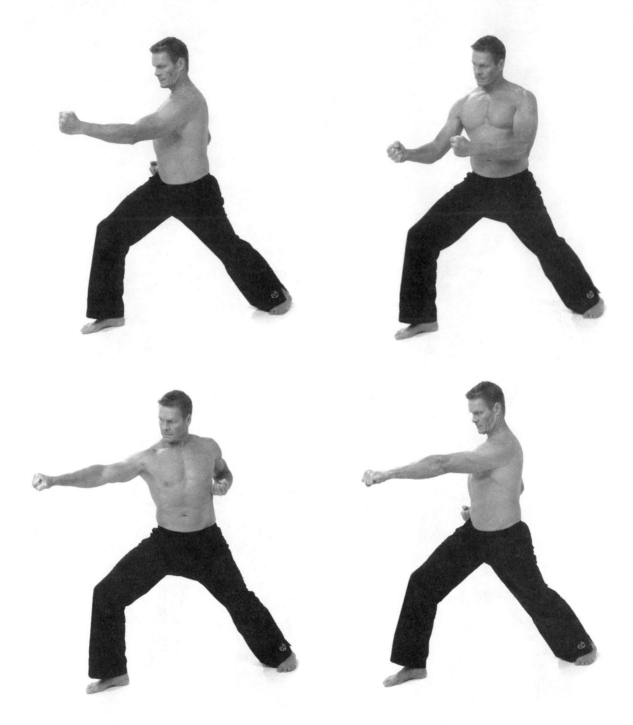

FIGHTING WARRIOR
FW15

Mark Divine and Catherine Divine

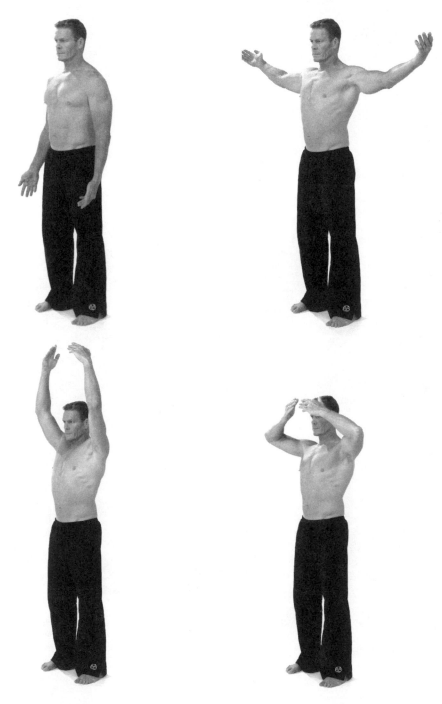

BRINGING DOWN THE HEAVENS
FW16

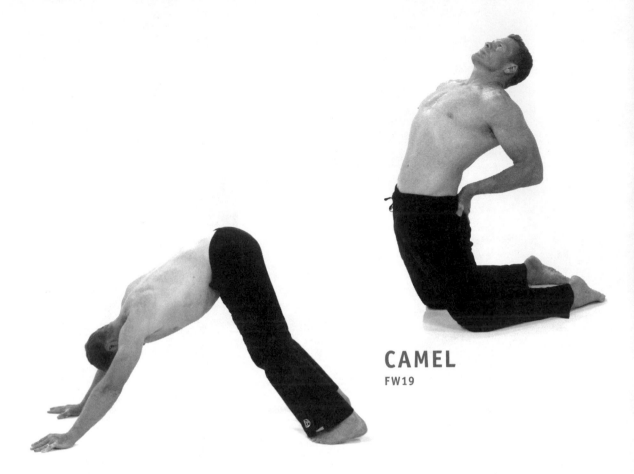

CAMEL
FW19

DOWN DOG
FW17

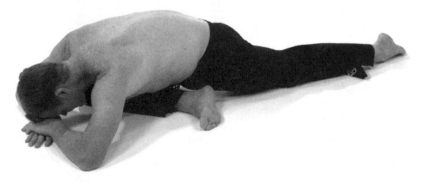

PIGEON
FW18

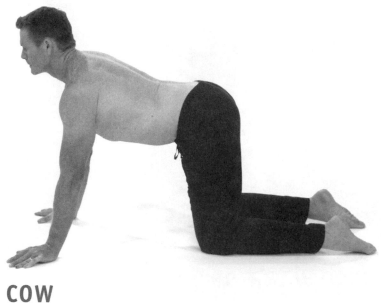

COW
FW20

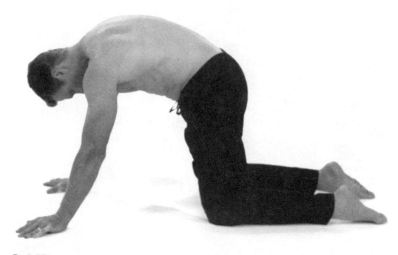

CAT
FW20

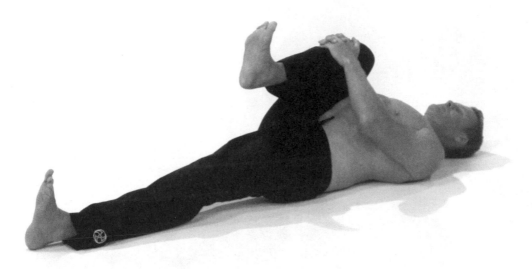

CLEANSING WARRIOR
FW21

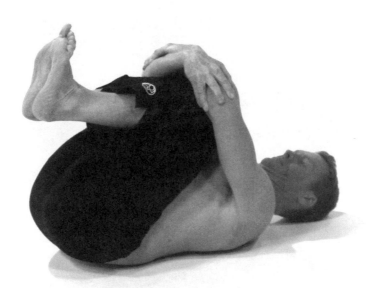

HEALTHY WARRIOR
FW22

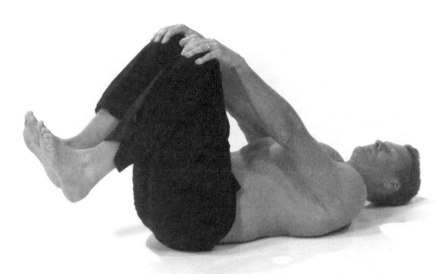

BACK ALIGNMENT
FW22

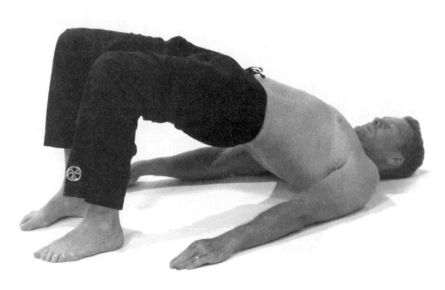

BRIDGE
FW23

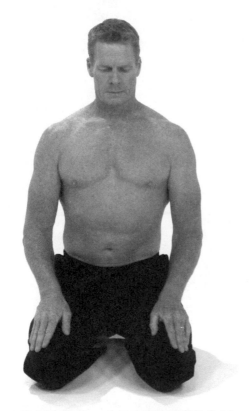

RESTING POSE
FW24

SEATED MEDITATION
FW25

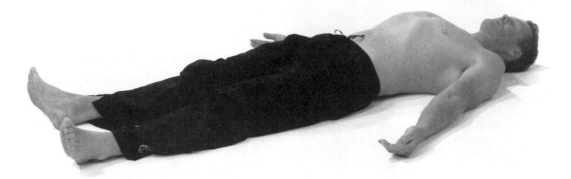

BOX
BREATHING
3-6-6-3 5X

**BOX BREATHING
3-6-6-3 5X**
FW26

Fighting Warrior

This sequence is about 45 minutes to an hour long and is as challenging as the Fit Warrior but differs in that it uses combat conditioning movements instead of functional exercises for the exercise part. This allows us to get a great "cardio" workout while practicing our strikes and kicks. (See the appendix for a description of the fight moves.) This sequence is excellent for anyone with fighting skills, or who enjoys cardio kickboxing.

You will bring a fighting-warrior attitude, as if you were in a sensitive situation and you will need to "bring it" to solve it. Visualizing an opponent during the sequences develops our visual acuity. As with Fit Warrior, there are two ways to perform this sequence type. The first is to sprinkle in the fight moves between the yoga poses, and the second is to do the standing poses to warm up, then do the fight sequences altogether, and finally finish with the seated poses. Both are equally effective, but the first keeps your heart rate down in an endurance training zone, while the latter ramps it up to an intensity zone. Choose whichever suits your needs and get busy! You don't need to be an experienced martial artist to have a blast with this sequence.

BOX
BREATHING
5X5

SUN
SAL
A

BOX BREATHING 5X5
FGW1

SUN SALUTATION A
FGW2

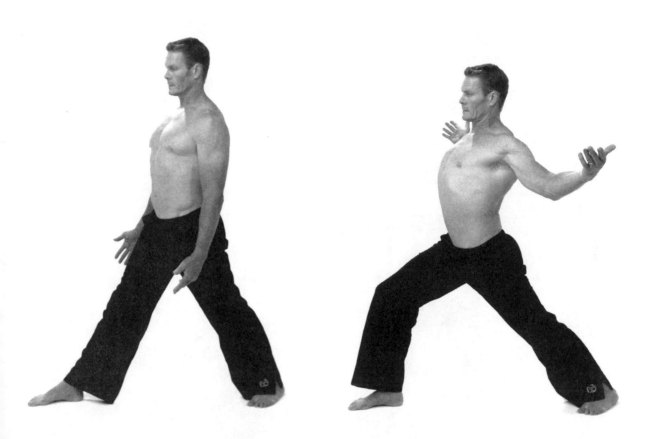

WARRIOR 1 WITH BREATH

FGW3

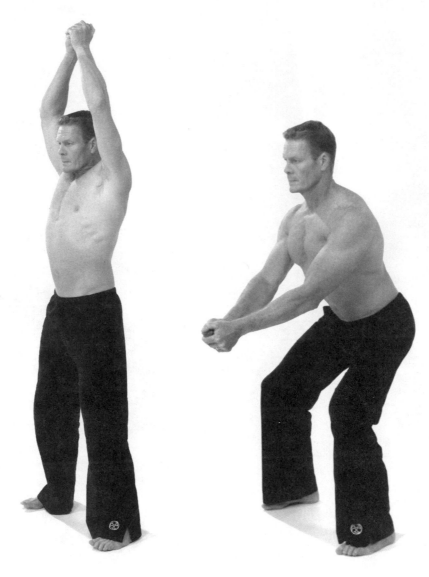

CHOPPING WOOD

FGW4

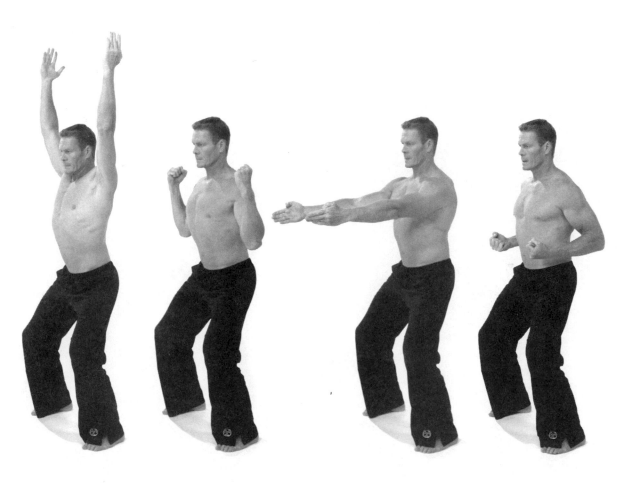

WARRIOR BREATH—100X
FGW5

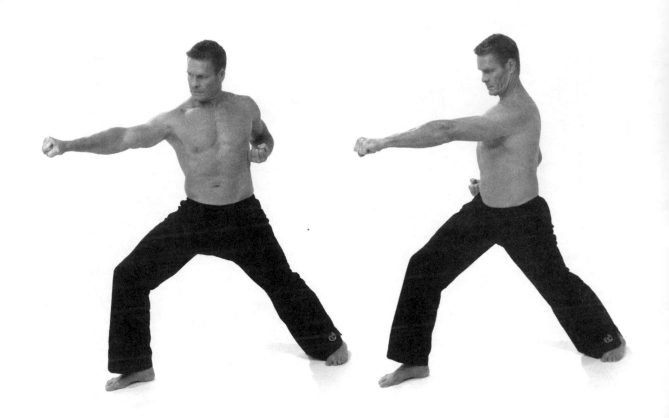

PUNCHING WARRIOR—20X EACH SIDE

FGW6

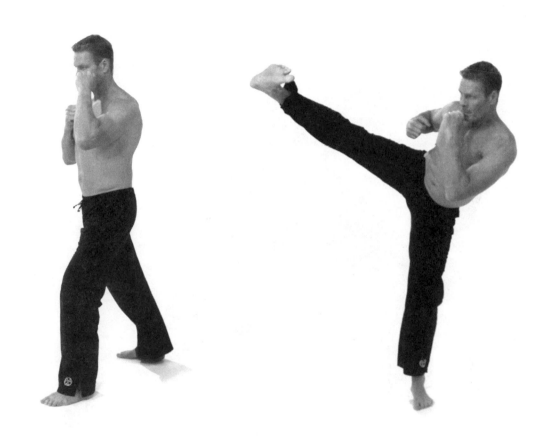

KICKING WARRIOR—20X EACH SIDE
FGW7

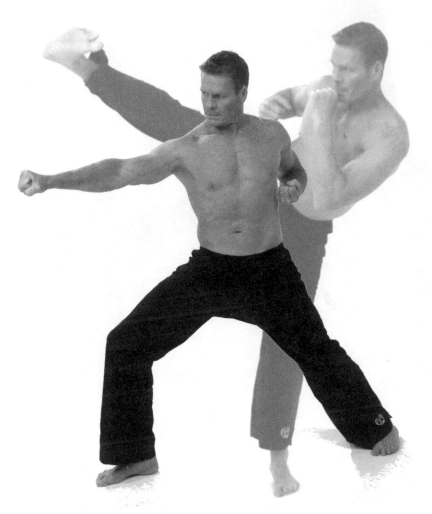

COMBINATION MODULE OF KICK AND PUNCH—20X EACH SIDE
FGW8

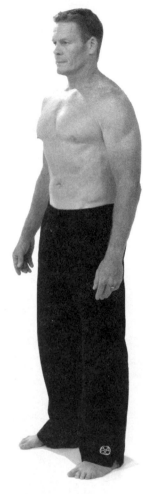

MOUNTAIN POSE— 5 BREATHS
FGW9

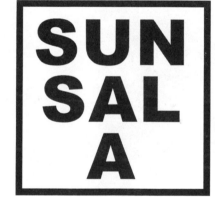

SUN SALUTATION A
FGW10

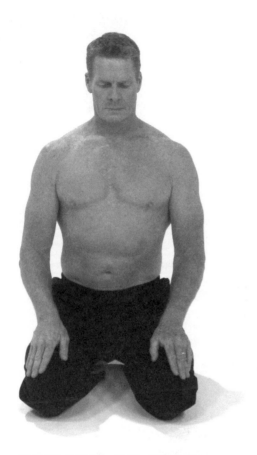

BREATH OF FIRE
FGW11

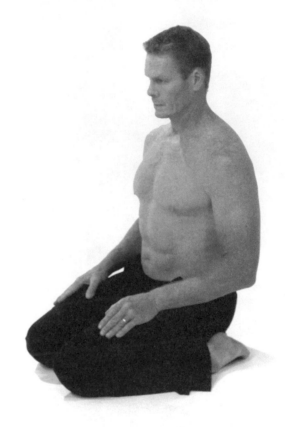

VICTORIOUS WARRIOR VISUALIZATION—EITHER STANDING OR SITTING
FGW12

Jedi Warrior

This sequence is 20 minutes long utilizing breathing and movements from the Chinese "warrior-yoga" art of Qigong, with select poses to support joint mobility and structure, while also enhancing our energetic body's health. Like many martial arts, we will experience this work at the physical level before experiencing it at the subtle energy level. This sequence is great for internal organ health as well as muscular strength and conditioning. Over time this sequence will train deeper awareness, and the attitude is that of one seeking mastery, much like the Jedi Knight training of Luke Skywalker in the movie *Star Wars*.

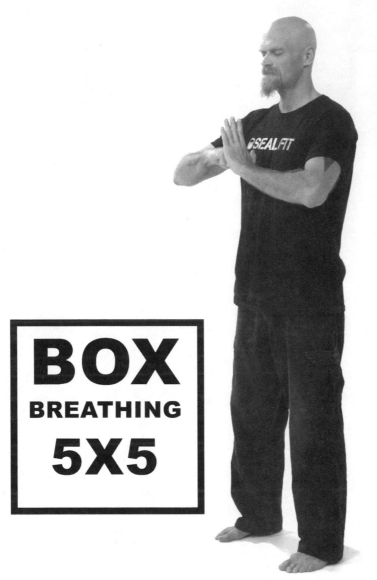

BOX BREATHING 5X5

BREATHING

5X5

BOX BREATHING 5X5—SET INTENTION
JW1

ROM DRILLS

ROM DRILLS
JW2

SUN SAL AX2

SUN SALUTATION A—2X
JW3

SUN SAL BX2

SUN SALUTATION B—2X
JW4

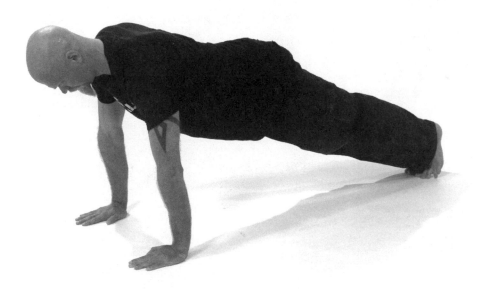

PLANK—HOLD FOR 30 SECONDS
JW5

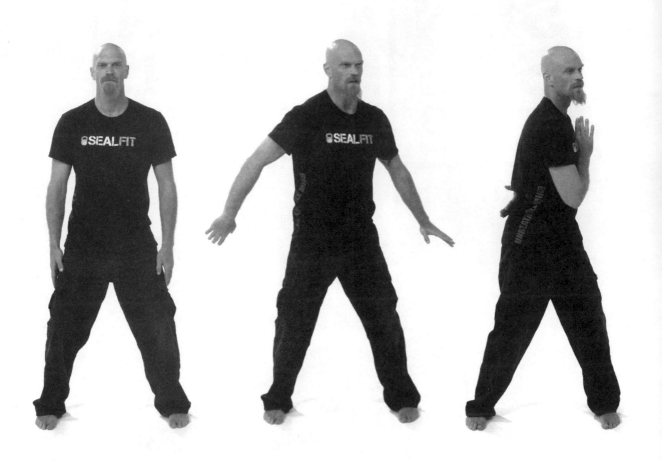

WINDMILL
JW6

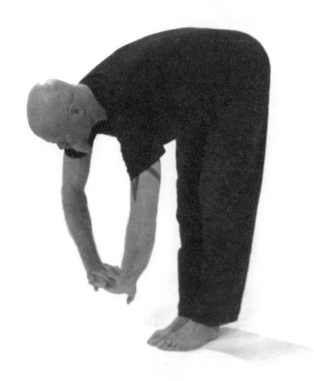

QIGONG OR "WATER MILL" FORWARD FOLD—3 MINUTES

JW7

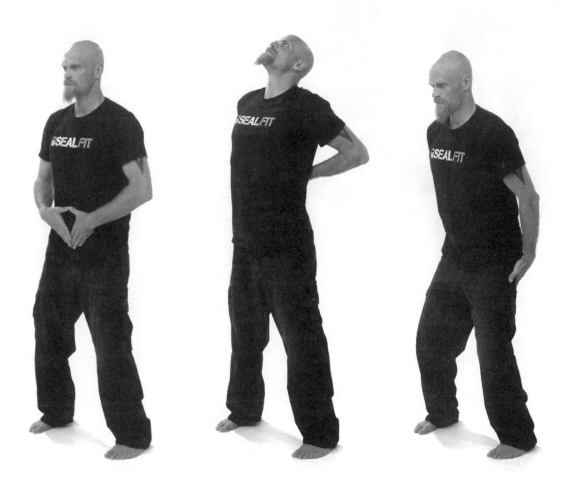

KI-UB
JW8

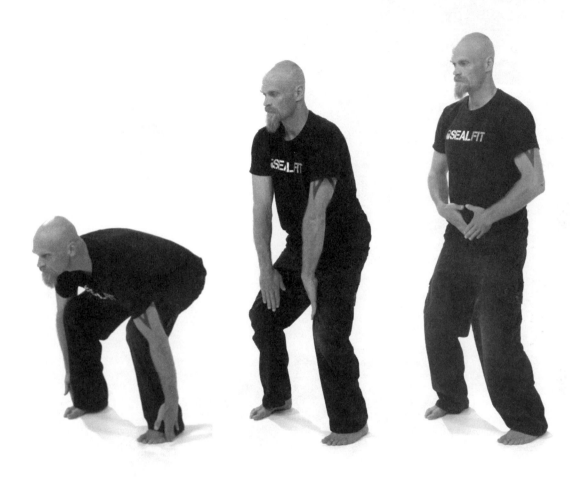

JW8

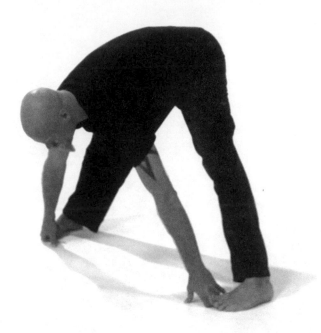

WIDE ANGLE FORWARD FOLD
JW9

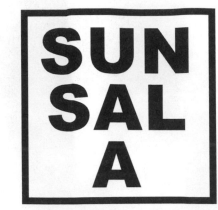

SUN SALUTATION A
JW10

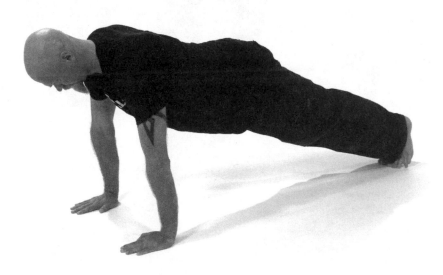

PLANK—HOLD FOR 1 TO 3 MINUTES
JW11

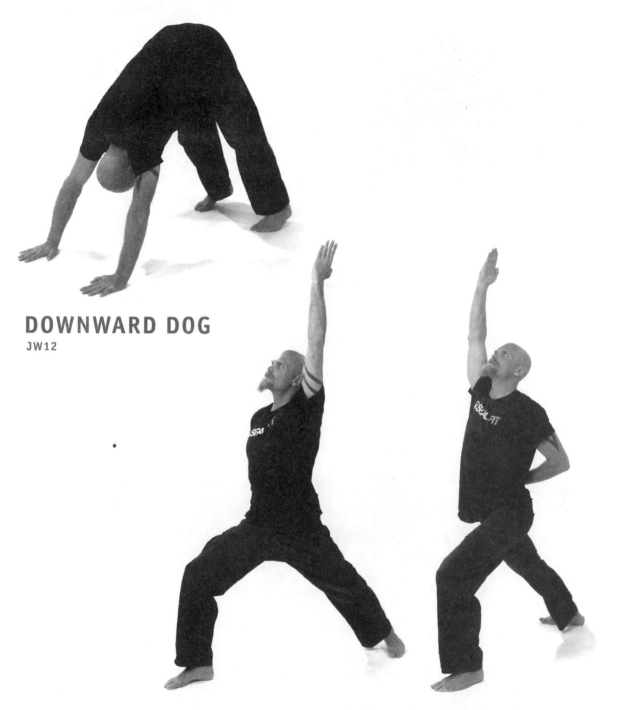

DOWNWARD DOG
JW12

EXALTED WARRIOR—EACH SIDE
JW13

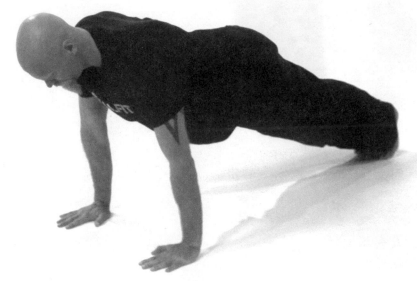

JW14

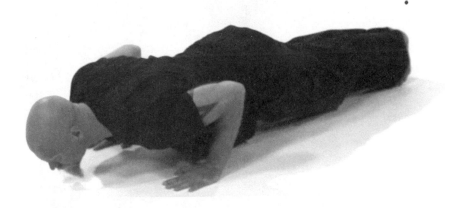

PUSH-UP—HOLD FOR 5 BREATHS

JW15

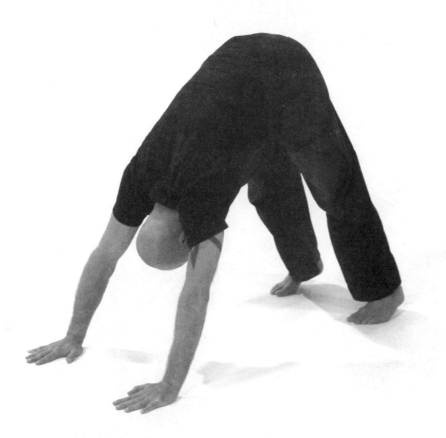

DOWNWARD DOG
JW16

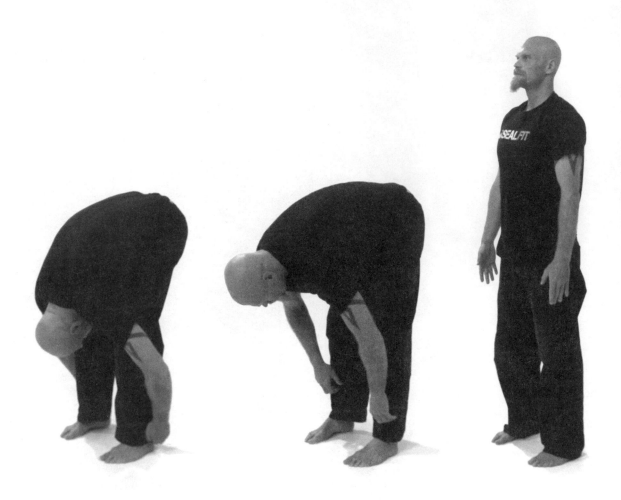

FORWARD FOLD—5 BREATHS—ROLL UP TO STANDING

JW17

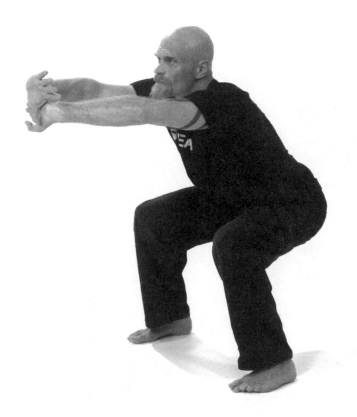

HORSE STANCE—HOLD FOR 3 TO 5 MINUTES
JW18

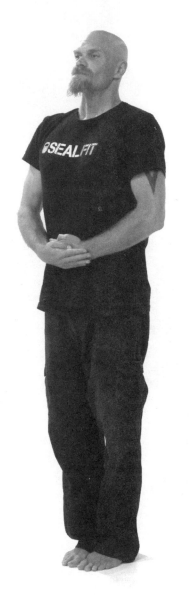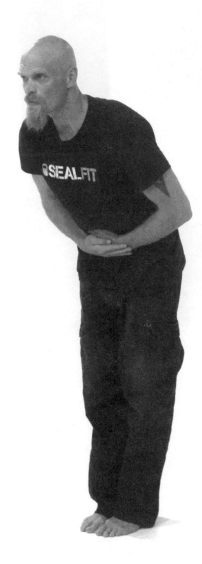

9 BREATHS—3 SETS

1. RELAX

2. SELF-HEALING VISUALIZATION

3. GRATITUDE

JW19

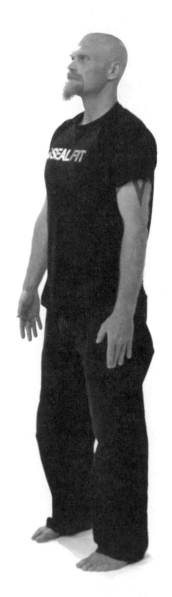

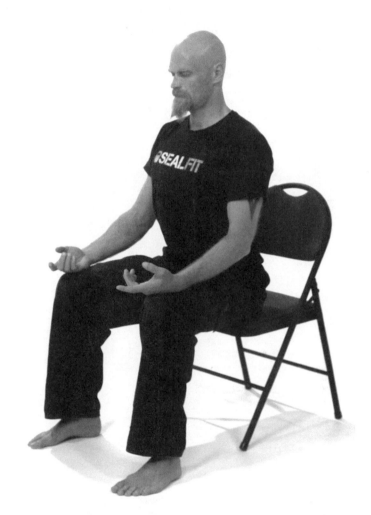

MOUNTAIN POSE—
REVISIT INTENTION
JW20

SEATED OR STANDING
MEDITATION—JEDI
WARRIOR VISUALIZATION
JW21

Ageless Warrior

This sequence is a comprehensive and balanced series of poses designed to optimize spinal and energetic health for longevity. *The focus is vitality, balance, and inspiration.* The universality of being ageless is to embody devotion to a greater cause than oneself, focus to execute tasks at any phase of life, and gratitude for the challenges and blessings that life brings to one as they walk the path of a warrior. Do this sequence once or twice a week and use the future me visualization to help you move toward your ageless self.

BOX BREATHING 1-2-2-1 5X

BOX BREATHING
—1:2:2:1 (5X)
AW1

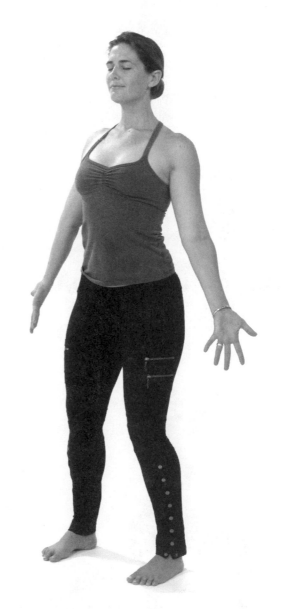

OPENING THE BOOK OF WISDOM (WHILE IN MOUNTAIN POSE)
AW2

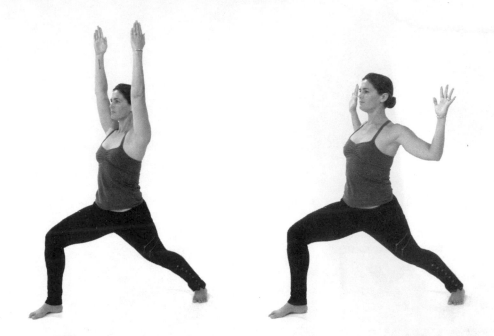

WARRIOR 1 WITH BREATH 5X

AW3

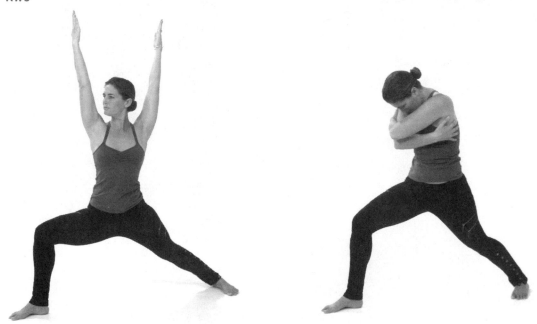

WARRIOR 2 WITH BREATH 5X
(ARMS STRAIGHT BY EARS)

AW4

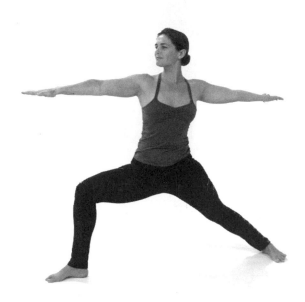

WARRIOR 2
(WITH BACK PALM UP)
AW5

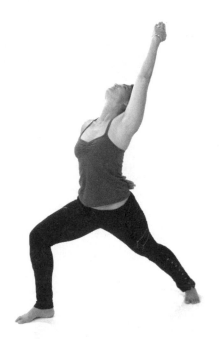

EXALTED WARRIOR
AW6

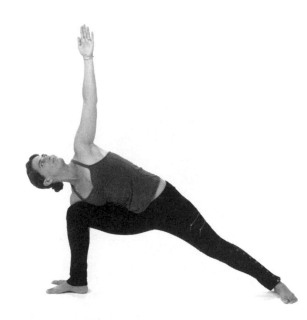

SIDE ANGLE POSE
AW7

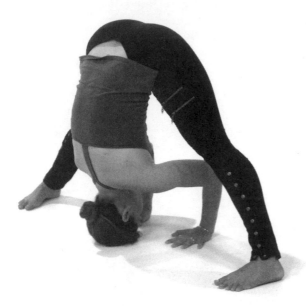

WIDE ANGLE POSE (TRANSITION TO OTHER SIDE AW1–AW8)

AW8

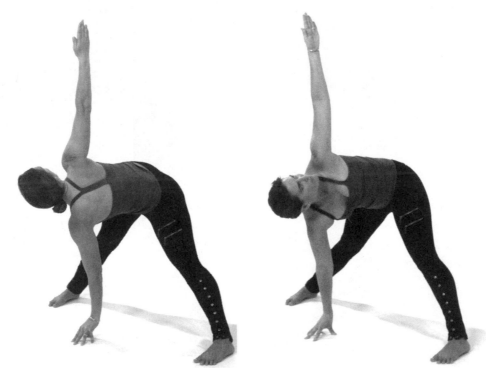

TWISTED WIDE ANGLE

AW9

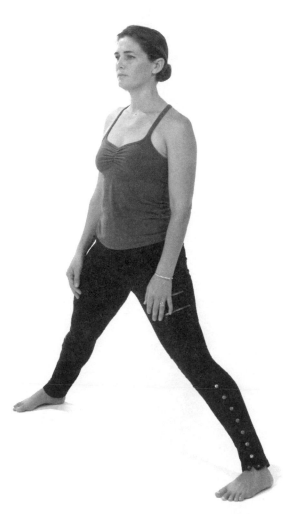

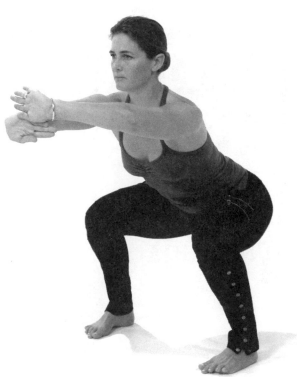

ROLL UP TO STANDING
AW10

HORSE STANCE—HOLD FOR 1 MINUTE
AW11

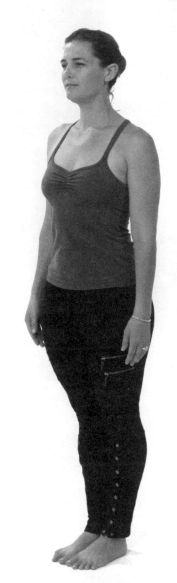

SUN SAL A

SUN SALUTATION A
AW12

STANDING MEDITATION WITH FUTURE SELF IN PERFECT HEALTH VISUALIZATION
AW13

Recovering Warrior (PTSD)

This sequence is a 15-minute restorative practice with a heavy focus on breathing, imagery, and holding select poses for a long time. The practice is designed to restore balance to the nervous system and calm an agitated mind. The mental attitude and imagery is one of total health and healing of the body, mind, and spirit. Performing one of the meditation or visualization practices immediately after this sequence is important.

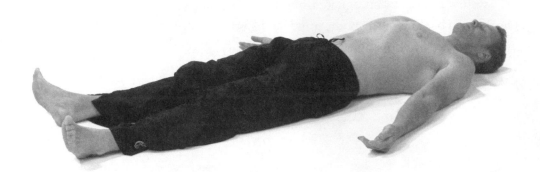

RESTING POSE—1:2 OR 4:8 BREATH (10X)
RW1

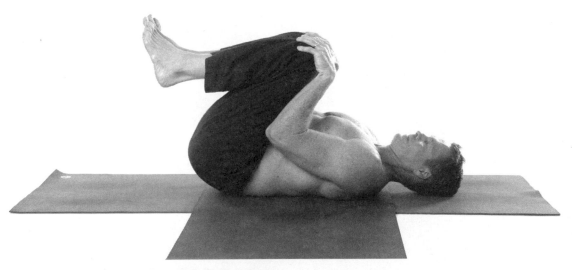

CLEANSING WARRIOR
RW2

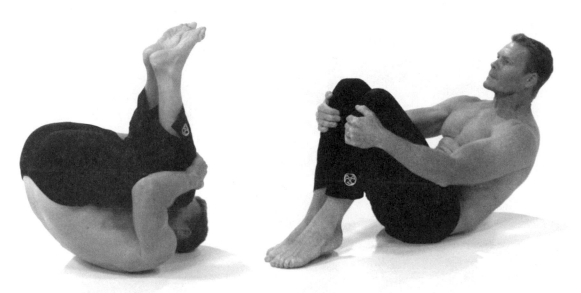

ROCK BACK AND FORTH 3X TO ENERGIZE YOUR SPINE

RW3A

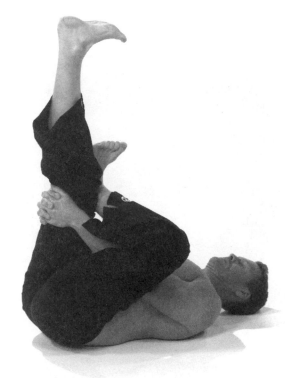

RECLINED PIGEON— EACH SIDE

RW3B

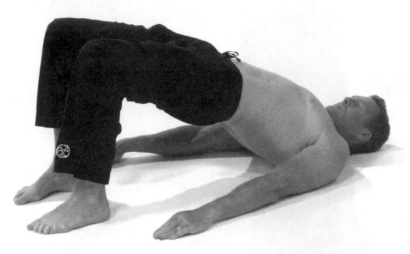

BRIDGE
RW4

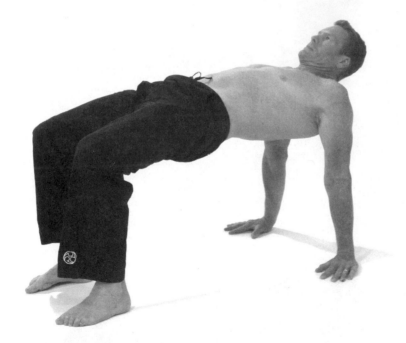

TABLETOP
RW5

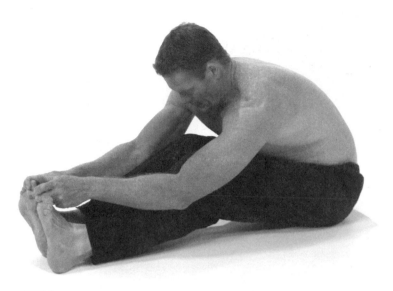

RW6A

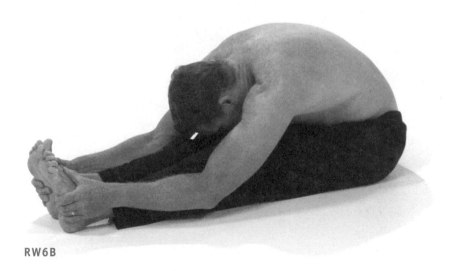

RW6B

SEATED FORWARD FOLD

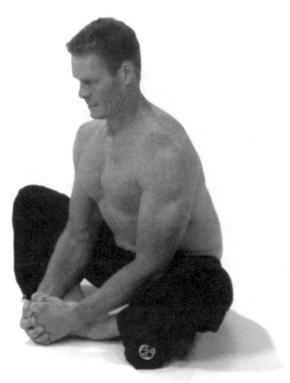

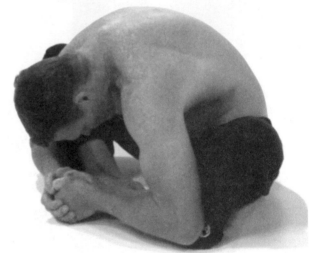

BUTTERFLY 1
RW7

BUTTERFLY 2
RW8

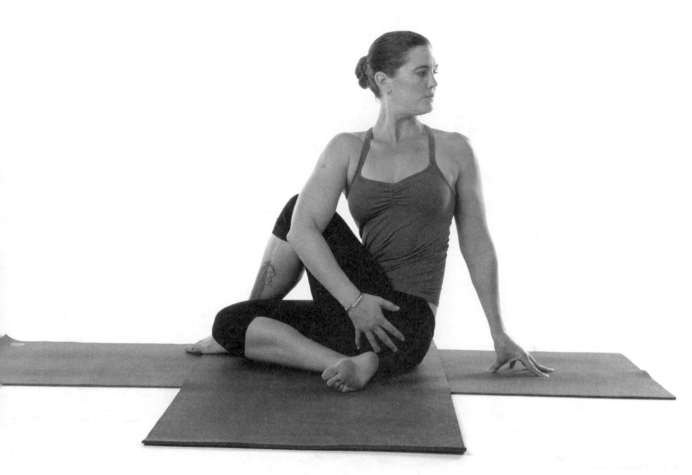

WISE WARRIOR—EACH SIDE
RW9

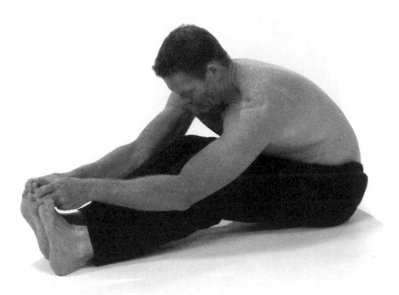

RW10A

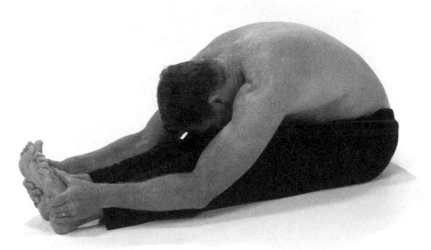

RW10B

SEATED FORWARD FOLD

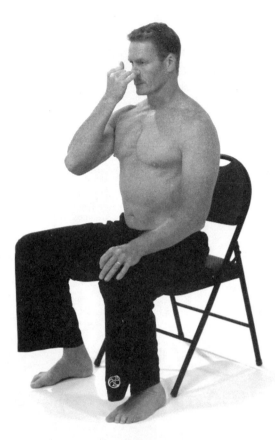

SEATED MEDITATION WITH ALTERNATE NOSTRIL BREATHING
RW11

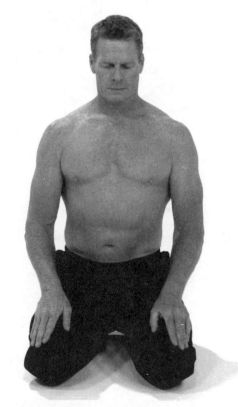

STILL WATER VISUALIZATION, FOLLOWED BY "FUTURE ME" IN PERFECT HEALTH
RW12

Hip Mobility Drill

This sequence focuses on opening the hips, twisting the spine, and engaging the core to provide stability in the pelvic region. It is particularly useful if you have been hiking or rucking for long distances, or done any weighted squatting.

Each pose will be held for 3 to 5 breaths.

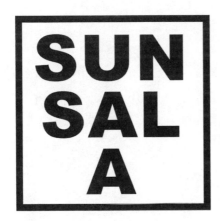

**SUN SALUTATION A
UNTIL DOWNWARD DOG**
RIGHT SIDE FIRST
HMD1

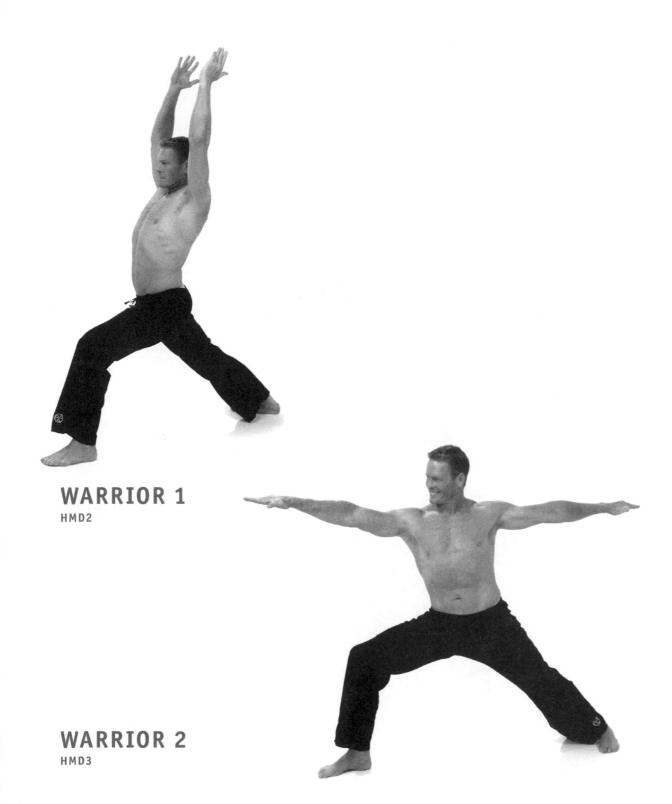

WARRIOR 1
HMD2

WARRIOR 2
HMD3

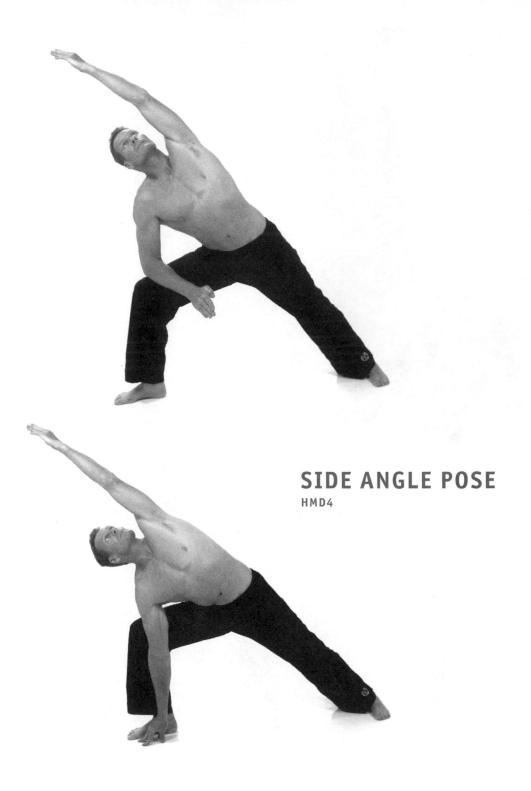

SIDE ANGLE POSE
HMD4

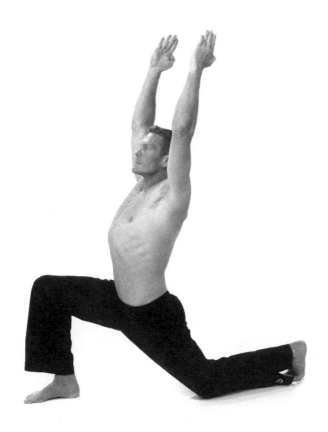

KNEELING WARRIOR, AKA ARCHER POSE
HMD5

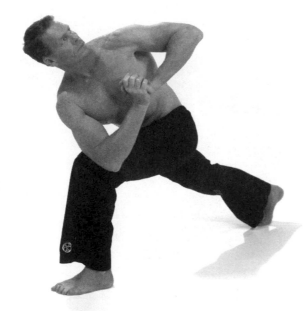

TWISTING WARRIOR
HMD6

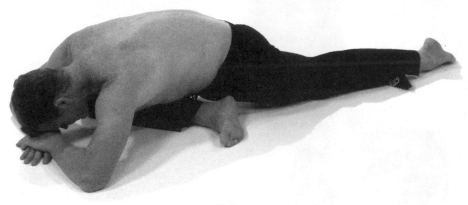

OR

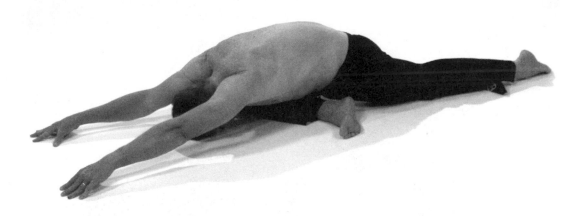

PIGEON
HMD7

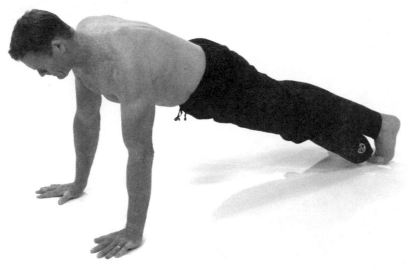

PLANK
HMD8

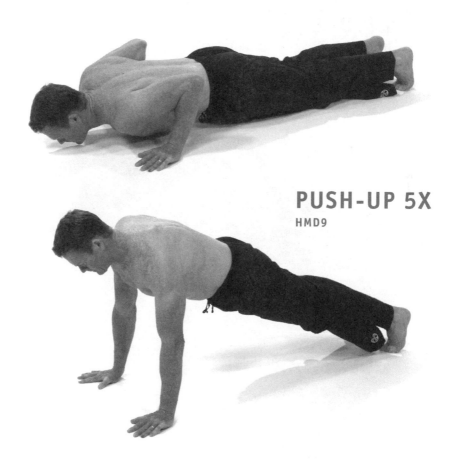

PUSH-UP 5X
HMD9

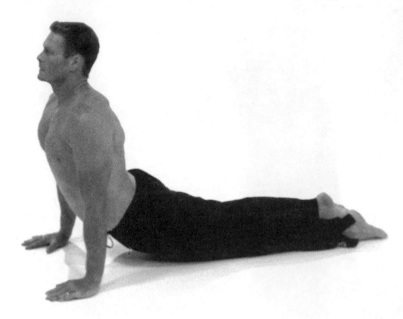

UP DOG
HMD10

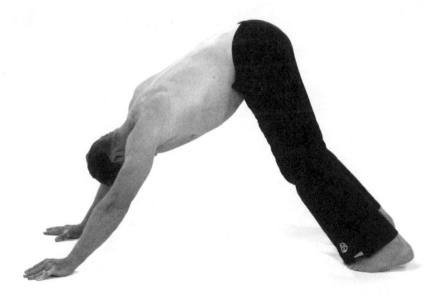

DOWNWARD DOG
REPEAT ON LEFT SIDE
HMD11

Meditation and Visualization Practice

Meditation is a key tactic in Kokoro Yoga. The overall progression of the training is meant to take you from the outer, externally focused physical level to the energetic, more internally focused breath/prana level, and finally into the deep interior of your heart-mind through meditation and visualization. These two practices are closely related working hand in glove to develop your mind and access your heart for optimal performance and growth.

Let's discuss meditation in more detail. Many in the West think meditation is just sitting quietly on a mat with eyes closed, or chanting a mantra. Another popular view is to follow a guided visualization using a CD or an app. These are valuable practices, for sure, but they represent the very beginning of your work. Ultimately meditation is a broad term for how we can use our inner mental skills to develop our heart-mind to better see truth, access wisdom, and experience love. There is a definite process to this though.

As mentioned earlier, the first step in the process is to deepen your concentration skills. Concentration is developed through the sequence practice, through breath control training, and through a practice whereby you deeply concentrate on one thing, such as an object or symbol. The object of focus can be external, such as a candle, a symbol like a cross, or an image like a yantra or mandala or a sunset. The object of focus can also be internally generated, such as focusing on the movement of breath, a count, sound, mantra, prayer, koan (thought question), scriptural verse, poem, or image. The best idea is to just choose something that is easy for you to focus on and deeply meaningful. The point of concentration practice is to train your thinking mind to be still. Over time you will be able to focus for long periods. This pays big dividends when it comes to achieving your goals in life. Concentration practice requires a deliberate effort and is typically done after a movement practice or as a stand-alone event.

As your concentration deepens, so does your awareness of what is going on around you and inside of you. You are now connecting to your perceiving mind, which knows without being taught something. Truth about nature is experienced through this part of your mind. The practice of mindfulness meditation is a nice tool to expand this growing awareness even more and to train your mind to click into a place of action instead of reaction. This technique can be used walking on the beach, washing dishes, or while shopping. It is a great way to extend your training throughout the day. The excuse of not having time to train falls apart when you consider that box breathing and mindfulness meditation can be performed almost anywhere and anytime.

Visualization is meditation with imagery that you create and direct. Visualizing Jesus Christ while you meditate is an example. With Kokoro Yoga we want to develop our visual acuity and create powerful visions of our desired future states and accomplishments. We also use visualization to practice skills or to heal a wound. The power of visualization is awesome when the mind has been trained to concentrate and be still.

Patanjali told us that the purpose of yoga is to develop control over your mind, so you can get control over your life. So after we can concentrate deeply and maintain presence, then what? Well, the mind will continue to grasp after material objects, concepts, beliefs, and desires. The grasper (us) gets confused with the thing being grasped and leads us continually to false identification with things we accomplish or things we think we control outside of ourselves, or those cherished beliefs we cling to. Identification with a career, spouse, role, fancy car, etc., are examples, and when they change, which is inevitable, we fall apart because we have identified with them as "us." But none of the external things are us, and none of the beliefs or internal patterns are us, either. This always leads to suffering of some form or another, because none of these things last forever, and none of them has anything to do with who we really are.

The mind truly is a wily trickster, though. This instrument of perception of ours tricks us into thinking it is the boss, when in fact it works for your deeper self, your witnessing soul-centered self (recall the bliss layer from chapter 3). Insight, or self-reflection meditation is our method to disentangle the grasper from that which is grasped, and to clarify the mind so that it reflects reality clearly while serving you without complaint. This method is to have you meditate on your patterns and behavior and to work relentlessly to align with your spirit. You will reflect daily in meditation on alignment with your ethical stand and disciplines (recall the Yamas and Niyamas). Slowly you will be firmly seated in the driver's seat, steering your mind relentlessly toward your eternal witness's vision for your life's purpose. Your ego will be in its rightful place, retaining its healthy, positive qualities, dropping the negative and needy grasping for control. This final stage of meditation is how we develop into higher stages of healthy, integrated consciousness.

Through meditation practice we move from distraction to attention and then attention to understanding completely that which we concentrate on. You become a scientist studying the inner workings of your own human nature, and as your mind penetrates the inner workings of your own nature you begin to understand all of human nature. Information is exchanged between you and your object of focus, whether that is an image of Christ or your own disruptive patterns and you crack open your innate, intuitive intelligence. This stage of your development will bring great clarity and peace.

Beginning Meditation Technique

To begin a meditation or visualization practice you can start with a simple breath awareness exercise. This can be done anywhere, at your desk or in bed when you wake up for instance. Simply close your eyes and pay attention to your breath for a few moments.

It is advisable to create a "sacred space" in your home where you can do your yoga training, especially the meditation part. Having this space and using it every day will help you to focus as you implement your personal practice. It will also help keep others in your family or tribe from distracting you (more on how to develop a personal practice in the last chapter).

When you "sit" for meditation it is important that your spine is erect and not compressed in any way. The easiest way to accomplish this is to sit on the edge of a chair. Many think that there is some magic to sitting cross-legged on the floor. Not so—the reason this was done was because there weren't many chairs around back in the day! If you do sit on the floor, then you can use a small zazen bench (which is what I use) or stack some pillows to sit on. To create the sacred feeling, it helps to create an "altar" of sorts with a meaningful picture and candle. Plenty of information is available on how to begin a meditation practice, so I won't belabor the point. Let's now take a glance at a few of the insight meditation practices.

Full-Body Scan Stress Reduction

Sit comfortably, with your spine erect in such a way that it's as if a balloon is attached to the dome of your skull with a string, gently lengthening your spine upward. Your eyes can either be open or softly closed. Take a series of slow, deep breaths, and perform a light scan from the top of the skull downward, imagining a tingling flow of energy that relaxes you. Starting with the forehead, relax each section of your head and body with light attention, breathing into the awareness and exhaling tension. In this way, relax the muscles of the face, the neck, and the shoulders, observing the tension melt and drip away. Move through your chest, your abdomen, your lower back, and pelvic girdle, through to your upper legs, knees, and then lower legs. Finish with a scan of your feet, both the tops and the arches, and finally, the toes. Pay attention to the state of peace, relaxation, and energy that is now moving through you and in tune with your slow, deep breathing. Your body is completely relaxed; your mind is completely relaxed. Note that this relaxation sequence can be used for each of the visualization and meditation practices.

Now picture yourself on a footpath that you've taken before, on a pristine, beautiful day, where you can feel the warmth of the sun on your face and the rustle of a breeze moving through your hair. Walk on the path and soak in the stunning beauty of the moment. Pause to pick up a rock from the path, bring it up to your nose, and smell the grounded earthiness of your path. Place it back down and continue walking around a bend where you see and hear a freshwater stream. Breathe in as you let your mind sink into the beauty and power of the pure blue water. Allow the stream to calm your mind, your spirit, your body. This will take you to a place (over a long consistent practice) of neutral, nonjudgmental observation. If a thought stirs, you greet it with, "Not here, not now," and allow it to float away. It's in this place that you feel the witness expand with bliss and gratitude, an immense connection to everything and everyone. You allow a moment to soak in this deep, all-powerful silence.

Future Me

With the future me exercise, you are going to project a vision of your ideal self, at a point in the future, to build upon the connection with the internal witness and also carve a track for the subconscious to follow. The subconscious domain of your being cannot tell the difference between a real or an actual experience, so the more acute detail and emotional intensity you can pack this visualization with, the more effective it will be. The task here it to cultivate a powerful image of who you intend to become—the warrior on the path of mastery, a year or several years down the road. The time really depends on where you are in your life. As an aspiring SEAL my future me visualization was 1 year out, when I earned the coveted SEAL Trident. Today my future me is 10 to 20 years out when I have fulfilled my current vision.

When your mind is focused, after a short box breathing or body scan practice, conjure up a vision of a future version of yourself in the process of fulfilling your life purpose, or a momentous goal. You know that you have made it, having achieved a dream that required massive and dedicated action. You see it in full color with as much detail as possible, with real emotion. In this inner space you feel a humble acceptance, knowing you have aligned with your spirit and served a greater good. You're living in a highly tuned state of health and energy, and the goodness of the moment circulates with your blood. You feel fantastic and alive. This is the new you, now. Remain here for at least 5 minutes living the vision of your future self.

Returning your attention to the breath, experience the grace of the moment with humble gratitude. You return to the present moment, opening your eyes, highly energized, confident, at peace, with all your senses firing, and with the imbedded sense of having accomplished something worthwhile and important.

Grounding

Starting out in a comfortable seat with your eyes closed, gaze softly within. The spine is in alignment and the core is engaged. There is a softness and relaxation in the jaw and shoulders, as you sit upright and engaged. Begin to tune your awareness to the breath. Notice how it feels to breathe in and out through the nose. Notice if there is more ease when you inhale or exhale. You are just noticing, not judging or trying to change anything. Now begin to intentionally smooth out the edges of the breath, match the length of inhale and exhale to a count of 5 on each side so that 1 round of breath takes 10 seconds. Focus on this until it feels natural and you are in a state of relaxation and expanded awareness. Now connect to the area in the pelvic floor and the base of the spine. Take a few conscious breaths into your pelvic bowl and begin to visualize a bright red ball of energy that is glowing and radiating healing. Visually create roots growing from this ball the width of your torso down into the earth. Allow the roots with each breath to grow deeper and deeper into the earth until you have reached the core center of this planet and hook into it. Breathe gently into your roots. Then like you would drink through a straw to sip liquid, start to sip in the earth energy through the roots you have created. Allow the earth's energy to be drawn up into your body filling you with strength and vitality. See the origin of your roots as this glowing red orb get brighter and brighter as you recharge your body.

This is a meditation exercise you can also do standing barefoot in the park or on a beach or a mountain. It may also be used for curing issues like fatigue, depression, lethargy, and for times when you feel out of sorts or not yourself.

Willpower

Find a quiet place where you can settle into a comfortable seat. Your eyes can be open or closed. If the eyes are open, then keep a very soft gaze; maybe light a candle and gaze at the flame. If the eyes are closed, gaze inward and down toward the tip of the nose to assist in concentration. Place both hands over your belly and breathe into the belly expanding it out like a balloon and then exhale out through the mouth releasing tension. Inhale into the belly expanding it out and then exhale through the mouth expunging negative attitudes and thoughts. Inhale one more time into the belly expanding it out and then exhale out through the mouth with an ahhh sound, releasing unconscious thoughts that are not serving you well. You do not need to know what the tension or the thoughts are; the intention of letting go is enough. Relax your hands and place them palms down on your knees. Begin to breathe in and out through the nose at a natural pace. Now focus on your own internal energetic fire that is constantly burning off toxins as well as driving your will to be present and put forth effort in the world. Ask yourself: What is my purpose? As the answer arises, connect with your willpower energy in the belly and begin to fuel your purpose from this place of focus and passion. Anchor your purpose into the fire within and remain seated for a few more minutes in silence. Breathe with an awareness on your belly and the power that resides within.

Compassion

Lying flat on your back, place your right hand on your belly and your left hand on your heart center. Close your eyes softly and begin to tune into the frequency of your energetic heart center. This center traditionally is the place of universal love and compassion. Feel the physical heart beat in the belly and the heart regions. Turn your focus to the energy of your heart, in the center of your chest, and connect the energy of your breath with the vibration of your heart and feel as if your physical body is beginning to melt like snow in a warming sun. As the physical body softens and begins to let go of attachments relax the arms beside the body. Now ask the heart center: *What am I holding onto that no longer serves me?* As the question is answered let go of the story around the event, the person, or yourself and how any pain came to be. Just sit in the knowledge that holding on to negative emotions only restricts us from thriving at optimal levels.

With this attitude say to yourself 3 times in silence: *I now release _____ with love and acceptance. I acknowledge that _____ served its purpose for my growth and evolution.* Once you are finished with this affirmation begin to envision a ball of light glowing in your heart center. Breathe with the new awareness of compassion and love that you and everything is perfect right now in this moment. Feel your heart energy expand as you breathe compassion into your heart. Envision this glowing ball of light energy begin to spread through your entire body as you breathe naturally and with ease. If any resistance arises during the process and you notice any negative thoughts creeping in, interdict them with the statement: *This is a thought, it is not who I am.* Then move back into the visualization and continue to breathe for 5 more minutes with an open heart and a calm body and mind. When you are finished, sit up gently and bring your hands to your heart thanking it for its wisdom.

Sequence Appendix for Reference

1. PEACEFUL WARRIOR—MOST POSTURES HELD OR SEQUENCED THROUGH 5–10 BREATHS

PW1: Seated Meditation—Nostril Breathing

PW2: Alternate Nostril Breathing—Start inhale on left side, equal part count on inhale and exhale, retain breath at equal part count after inhale. Example: inhale through left nostril, close both nostrils retain, exhale right, inhale right nostril, close both nostrils retain, exhale left. Repeat for 7–14 rounds ending on exhale through the left nostril.

PW3: Cow Pose—Inhale

PW4: Cat Pose—Exhale

PW5: Child's Pose—Move into on exhale

PW6: Transition through to Cow—Move through on inhale

PW7: Down Dog—Move into on exhale

PW8: Kneeling Warrior Each Side—Move into on inhale, transition back to Down Dog on exhale

PW9: Wide Angle Forward Fold—Move into on exhale

PW10: Roll up to standing while exhaling

PW11A: 3 Part Movement Bringing Down the Heavens: 1. Inhale arms out and up, 2. continue to inhale as you lift heels and interlace fingers, 3. Exhale lower arms back alongside.

PW11B: Sun Salute A 2X

PW12: Warrior 1: Move into on Inhale

PW13: Warrior 2: Move into on Inhale

PW14: Side Angle Pose: Move into on Exhale

PW15: Exalted Warrior: Move into on Exhale

PW16: Plank: Move into on Inhale

PW17: Push-up: Move into on Exhale

PW 18: Upward Facing Dog: Move into on Inhale

PW19: Downward Facing Dog: Move into on Exhale; Repeat on Left Side

PW 20: Sharp Warrior: Move into on Exhale

PW 21: Sun Salute A

PW 22: Tree Pose: Move into on Inhale

PW 23: Dancer: Move into on Inhale

PW 24: Sun Salute A as a transition to seated position

PW 25: Seated Forward Fold: Move into on Exhale

PW 26: Table Top: Move into on Inhale

PW 27: Cleansing Warrior: Bring knees into chest on exhale inhale straighten arms and bring knees away from chest

PW 28: Bridge: Move into on Inhale

PW 29: Bridge or Wheel: Move into on Inhale

PW 30: Reclined Pigeon: Move into on Exhale

PW 31: Happy Baby Pose: Move into on Inhale

PW 32: Healthy Warrior: Move into on Exhale

PW 33: Butterfly 1&2: Move into on Exhale

PW 34: Reclined Warrior Pose: Move into on Exhale

PW 35: Resting Pose: Breathe at natural pace, let go of victorious breath or any counted breathing pattern.

PW 36: Seated Meditation—Focus on revisit intention/breath followed by compassion and peace meditation: Breathe at natural pace, let go of victorious breath or any counted breathing pattern.

2. ZEN WARRIOR—MOST POSTURES HELD OR SEQUENCED THROUGH 5–10 BREATHS

ZW1: Mountain Pose: Breathe with Focus

ZW 2: Sun Salute A 3x

ZW 3: Sun Salute B 3x

ZW 4: Brining Down the Heavens: 1. Inhale arms out and up, 2. continue to inhale as you lift heels and interlace fingers, 3. Exhale lower arms back alongside.

ZW 5: Kicking Warrior: Inhale in Warrior 1 then Move into kick on Exhale

ZW 6: Mountain Pose: Breathe with Focus

ZW 7: Archer Warrior: 1. Inhale in Warrior 2 bring back hand so palms face each other 2. Through a pinhole shape of the mouth exhale in spurts and as you pull back the metaphoric bow

ZW 8: Scooping the Moon: Move into on Inhale, Exhale as back of the hand returns to in front of forehead

ZW 9: Warrior Musashi: Move into on Inhale and Exhale Strike

ZW 10: Sun Salute A—Finish in Down Dog and come to knees

ZW 11: Camel: Move into on Inhale

ZW 12: Reclined Warrior Pose: Move into on Exhale

ZW 13: Wise Warrior Twist: Move into on Exhale and find length of spine on the Inhale

ZW 14: Rock back and forth to standing in mountain: Rock back on inhale and forward on exhale

ZW 15: Sun Salute A to push up lower on the belly

ZW 16: 1 Arm Locust: Move into on Inhale

ZW 17: Locust: Move into on Inhale

ZW 18: Bow: Move into on Inhale

ZW 19: Reverse Push-up: Move into on Inhale

ZW 20: 5x Push-up: Exhale as you lower

ZW 21: Up Dog or Cobra: Move into on Inhale

ZW 22: Grateful Warrior-Child's pose with palms up: Move into on Exhale

ZW 23: Cow: Move into on Inhale

ZW 24: Cat: Move into on Exhale

ZW 25: Seated Meditation position for Box breathing: Nostril breathing

ZW 26: Stay in Seated or come to Resting Pose for Grounding and strength meditation: Breathe at natural pace, let go of victorious breath or any counted breathing pattern.

3. FIT WARRIOR—MOST POSTURES HELD OR SEQUENCED THROUGH 5–10 BREATHS, WHEN IN FIT MODULE THEN EACH MOVEMENT IS DONE ON AN INDIVIDUAL BREATH

FW 1: Box Breathing: Nostril breathing

FW 2: Seated Meditation: Breathe at natural pace, let go of victorious breath or any counted breathing pattern.

FW 3: Cat/Cow: Cow on Inhale and Move into on Exhale

FW 4: Downward Facing Dog: Move into on Exhale after 5 breaths step feet forward

FW 5: Forward Fold come to standing

FW 6: Sun A 2x

FW 7: Sun B 2x

FW 8: Triangle: Move into on Exhale

FW 9: Twisted Triangle: Move into on Exhale

FW 10: Sharp Warrior: Move into on Exhale

FW 11: Wide Angle Forward Fold: Move into on Exhale

FW 12: Wide Angle Twist: Move into on Exhale, when complete on both sides come to mountain

FW13: Fit Module x3

FM1: Burpees, bring hands to floor

FM2: Jump back to plank position

FM3 AND 4: Push up

FM5: Jump Forward

FM6: Jump up and clap hands overhead

FM7: Jumping squats, go into squat position, knees track over toes and the weight in heels

FM8: Jump up and land back in squat to repeat

FM9: Mountain Climbers, plank position and jump on foot forward to outside of hand

FM10: Engaging core jump leading foot back as the back foot comes forward, count of 4 for 1 count of mountain climbers

FM11: Flutter kicks, laying on back with palms on ground while hands are supporting back, chest is lifted, legs hovering a few inches above the ground, lift one leg higher to start

FM12: as the leading leg lifts the other leg lowers slightly, count of 4 for 1 count of flutter kicks

FM13: Sit-Ups, start on your back with feet together hands overhead

FM14: With engaged abdominal muscles come up and touch your toes

FM15: Push-Ups, plank position inhale

FM16: Lower chest to ground on exhale, return to plank

FW14: Scooping the Moon: Move into on Inhale, Exhale as back of the hand returns to in front of forehead

FW15: Fighting Warrior-Punching: Inhale in Warrior and Exhale to punch

FW16: Bringing Down the Heavens: 1. Inhale arms out and up, 2. continue to inhale as you lift heels and interlace fingers, 3. Exhale lower arms back alongside.

FW17: Downward Facing Dog: Move into on Exhale

FW18: Pigeon: Move into on Exhale

FW19: Camel: Move into on Inhale

FW20: Cat/Cow: Cow on Inhale and Move into on Exhale

FW21: Cleansing Warrior: Move into on Exhale and start with right side

FW22: Healthy Warrior with movement: Move into on Exhale

FW23: Bridge: Move into on Inhale

FW24: Resting Pose: Breathe at natural pace, let go of victorious breath or any counted breathing pattern.

FW25: Seated Meditation: Breathe at natural pace, let go of victorious breath or any counted breathing pattern.

FW26: Box Breathing: Nostril Breathing

4. FIGHTING WARRIOR—MOST POSTURES HELD OR SEQUENCED THROUGH 5–10 BREATHS

FGW1: Box Breathing: Nostril Breathing

FGW2: Sun Salute A

FGW3: Warrior 1 with Breath: Start with arms alongside the body and Move into Warrior 1 with arms out to side and elbows bent, on Inhale

FGW4: Chopping Wood: Move into on Inhale and Chop on Exhale

FGW5: Warrior Breath 100x: Inhale arms up, exhale Pull arms down quickly, Inhale arms out in front, exhale arms in quickly. This is designed to build focus and heat.

FGW6: Punching Warrior 20x each side: Move into on Inhale, exhale punch

FGW7: Kicking Warrior 20x each side: Prep on inhale, Exhale kick

FGW8: Combination Module of kick on punch 20x each side: Prep on inhale, Exhale kick and punch

FGW9: Mountain Pose 5 breaths: Nostril Breathing

FGW10: Sun Salute A

FGW11: Seated Position with Breath of Fire: Inhale, Quick rapid Exhale as you pulse belly in and out

FGW12: Victorious Warrior Visualization seated or standing meditation

5. JEDI WARRIOR—MOST POSTURES HELD OR SEQUENCED THROUGH 5–10 BREATHS

JW1: Box Breathing and set intention: Nostril breathing

JW2: ROM Drills: Nostril breathing

JW3: Sun Salute A 2x

JW4: Sun Salute B 2x

JW5: Plank hold 30 seconds: Nostril breathing

JW6: Windmill: Start on Inhale the twist is on an Exhale

JW7: Qigong Forward Fold—Hold 3 minutes: Nostril Breathing

JW8: Ki Ub: Inhale as you Breathe into belly, Exhale as you bring hands to low back and then Inhale as you look up and Exhale as you bring hands down back of legs to the feet, Inhale as you bring hands up the calves and thighs and Exhale as the hands return back to the belly.

JW9: Wide Angle Forward Fold: Move into on Exhale

JW10: Sun Salute A to plank position

JW11: Plank hold for 1–3 minutes: Nostril breathing

JW12: Down Dog: Move into on Exhale

JW13: Exalted Warrior each side: Move into on Inhale

JW14: Plank: Move into on Inhale

JW15: Push-up: Move into on Exhale

JW16: Down Dog-walk feet forward: Move into on Exhale

JW17: Forward Fold-roll up to standing: Exhale as you roll up

JW18: Horse Stance: Move into on Exhale

JW19: 9 Breath—3 sets: Inhale as you lean back, Exhale as you fold torso forward

JW20: Mountain-Revisit intention: Nostril Breathing

JW21: Seated or Standing Meditation—Jedi Warrior Visualization: Breathe at natural pace, let go of victorious breath or any counted breathing pattern.

6. AGELESS WARRIOR—ALL POSTURES HELD OR SEQUENCED THROUGH 5–10 BREATHS

AW1: Box Breathing: Nostril breathing

AW2: Mountain Pose; Repeat 5x

AW3: Warrior 1 w/Breath Repeat 5x

AW4: Warrior 2: Arms straight by the ears: Move into on Inhale, Exhale round upper back and wrap arms around the body

AW5: Warrior 2: Back Palm Up: Move into on Exhale

AW6: Exalted Warrior: Move into on Exhale

AW7: Side Angle Pose: Move into on Exhale

AW8: Wide Angle Forward Fold: Move into on Exhale

AW9: Twisted Wide Angle Pose: Twist on Exhale

AW10: Roll up to Standing: Roll up on Exhale

AW11: Horse Stance: Move into on Exhale

AW12: Sun Salute A

AW13: Standing Meditation of Future Self in Perfect Health (option to do seated or in lying meditation form): Breathe at natural pace, let go of victorious breath or any counted breathing pattern.

7. RECOVERING WARRIOR (PTSD SUPPORT AND HEALING)—MOST POSTURES HELD OR SEQUENCED THROUGH 5–10 BREATHS

RW1: Resting Pose: Breathe at natural pace, let go of victorious breath or any counted breathing pattern.

RW2: Cleansing Warrior: Both knees come in on Exhale, Inhale straighten arms, Repeat 5x

RW3A: Rock Back and Forth 3x finish lying on back

RW3B: Reclined Pigeon Each Side: Move into on Exhale

RW4: Bridge: Move into on Inhale

RW5: Table Top: Move into on Inhale

RW6: Seated Forward Fold A and B: Move into on Exhale

RW7: Butterfly 1: Move into on Exhale

RW8: Butterfly 2: Move into on Exhale

RW9: Wise Warrior: Move into on Exhale

RW10: Seated Forward Fold A and B: Move into on Exhale

RW11: Seated Meditation with Alternate Nostril Breathing: Alternate Nostril Breathing— Start inhale on left side, equal part count on inhale and exhale, retain breath at equal part count after inhale. Example: inhale through left nostril, close both nostrils retain, exhale right, inhale right nostril, close both nostrils retain, exhale left. Repeat for 7–14 rounds ending on exhale through the left nostril.

RW12: Still Water Visualization

8. HIP MOBILITY DRILL—MOST POSTURES HELD OR SEQUENCED THROUGH 5–10 BREATHS

HMD1: Sun A until Down Dog

HMD2: Warrior 1: Move into on Inhale

HMD3: Warrior 2: Move into on Inhale

HMD4: Side Angle Pose: Move into on Exhale

HMD5: Kneeling Warrior: Move into on Inhale

HMD6: Twisting Warrior: Move into on Exhale

HMD7: Pigeon: Move into on Exhale

HMD8: from Down Dog Plank: Move into on inhale

HMD9: Push-up: Move into on Exhale

HMD10: Up Dog: Move into on Inhale

HMD11: Down Dog—Repeat on Left side and once finished with Left Side complete Sun A and return to standing

*For all sequences except the PTSD we encourage you to add inversions at the end before meditation if you have learned them from an instructor and feel safe at home to do them on your own. Poses encouraged if suitable are headstand, handstand, shoulder stand, forearm balance, and plow pose.

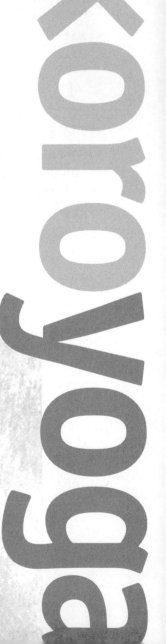

CHAPTER **6**

POSES AND MOVEMENTS

Yoga, an ancient but perfect science, deals with the evolution of humanity. This evolution includes all aspects of one's being, from bodily health to self-realization. Yoga means union—the union of body with consciousness and consciousness with the soul. Yoga cultivates the ways of maintaining a balanced attitude in day-to-day life and endows skill in the performance of one's actions.

—B. K. S. IYENGAR, *ASTADALA YOGAMALA*

CONSIDER THIS CHAPTER YOUR MASTER REFERENCE SOURCE FOR DETAILED INSTRUCTIONS AND PHOTOS FOR ALL KOKORO YOGA POSES AND MOVEMENTS PRESENTED IN THIS BOOK.

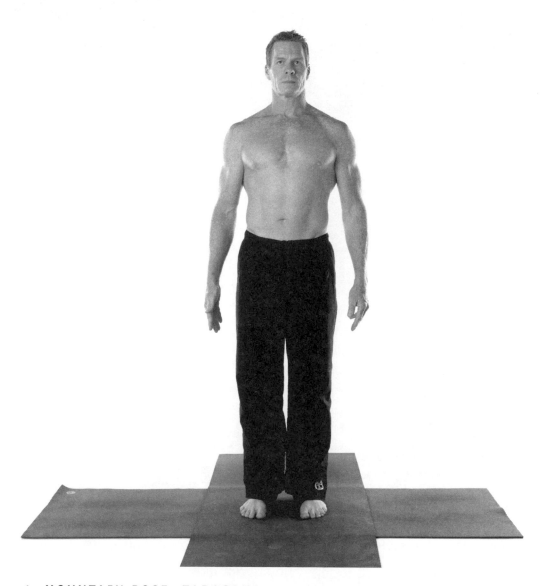

1. MOUNTAIN POSE—TADASANA

Standing with feet together or hip-width apart, the spine is in alignment and abdominals engaged. Shoulders are back and the chest is uplifted, the body is strong, and you are balanced on all four corners of your feet. This is the foundation for all standing poses.

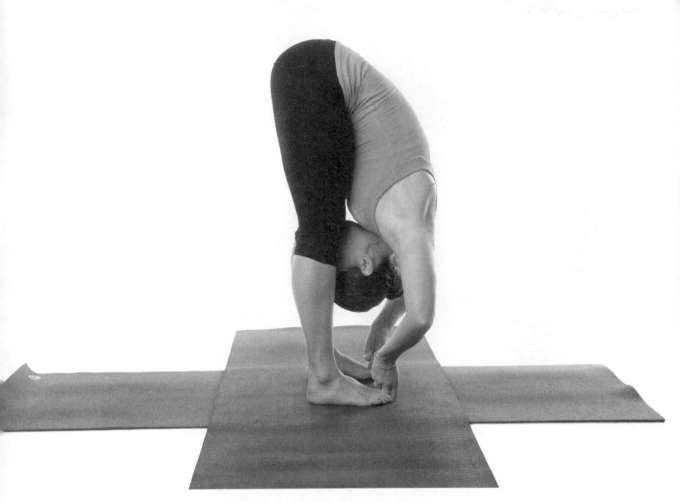

2. STANDING FORWARD FOLD—UTTANASANA

Stand with feet together or hip-width apart. Draw the belly button into the spine and engage quadriceps and abdominal muscles while folding forward. If you have lower-back issues, keep the knees slightly bent; otherwise maintain strong, straight legs with weight evenly distributed throughout the feet.

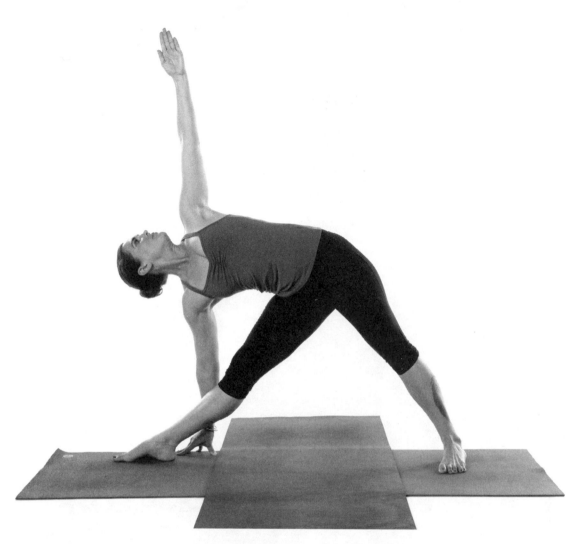

3. TRIANGLE POSE—TRIKONASANA

Feet are a minimum of 3 feet apart, with heels in alignment. Leading foot is open at a 90-degree angle, and the back foot at a 45-degree angle. Hips are open and all muscles of the body are engaged. Leading hand is on the floor, shin, or calf. The opposite arm is long and straight. Gaze is set at the fingertips.

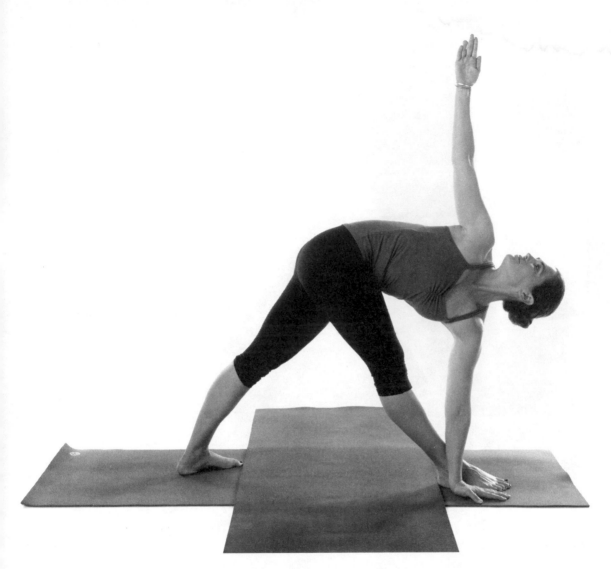

4.TWISTED TRIANGLE POSE—PARIVRTTA TRIKONASANA

Feet are at a minimum 3 feet apart with heels aligned. The leading foot is at 90 degrees and the back foot is at 65 degrees. Hips are aligned and the twist happens from the base of the spine through the top of the head. Leading arm is extended and straight in the air with eyes focused on fingertips. The opposite hand is on the outside of the leading foot or on the shin or thigh.

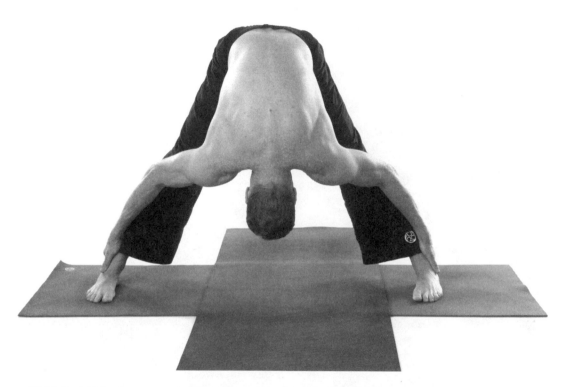

5. WIDE-ANGLE FORWARD FOLD—PRASARITA PADOTTANASANA

Feet are at 3 to 4 feet apart, heels slightly out, hands are on the floor between the feet, press into the outer edges of the feet, bring top of the head to the ground or a block, lift the sit bones toward the ceiling as you lift the kneecaps engaging the thighs.

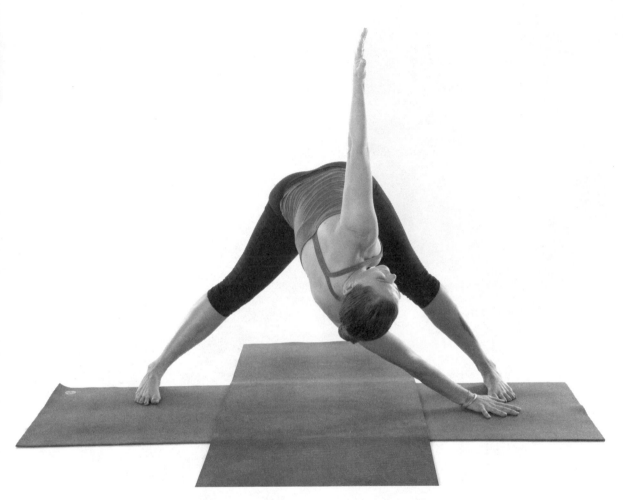

6. TWISTED FORWARD FOLD—PARIVRTTA PADOTTANASANA

Start with the Wide-Angle Forward Fold. Begin with left hand in the middle of the feet, twist torso bringing the right hand up toward the ceiling or on the sacrum, switch to other side.

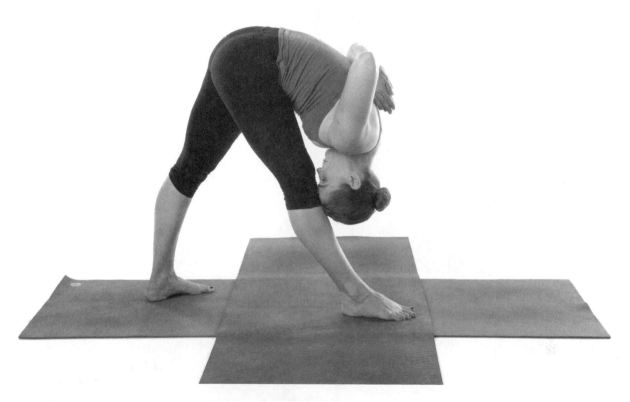

7. SHARP WARRIOR—PARSVAKONASANA

Feet are at a minimum 2.5 feet apart, leading foot is at a 90-degree angle, back foot is at a 65-degree angle, torso folds forward with an active or rounded spine, hips are aligned, hands are in prayer position between the shoulder blades with palms pressing together (or palms placed on the hips or floor for more balance). Bring the forehead to the knee or chin to shin, and gaze is at the tip of the nose.

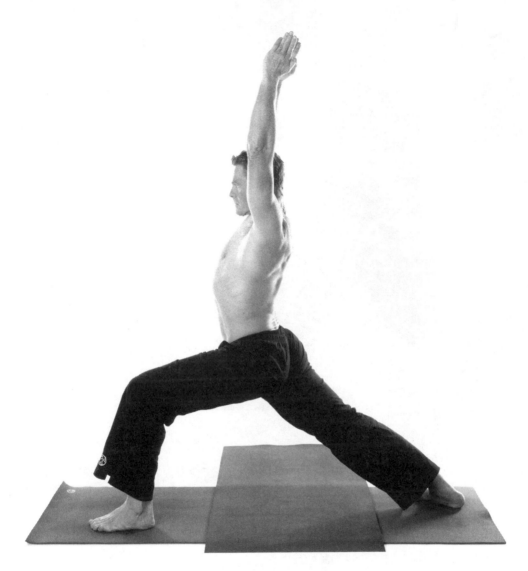

8. WARRIOR 1—VIRABHADRASANA A

Feet are at a minimum 3 feet apart with the leading foot at a 90-degree angle and the back foot at a 65-degree angle, hips are aligned and the leading leg is bent so that the thigh is parallel to the ground, the back leg is straight, torso is in a slight upper backbend, arms are lifted alongside the head, actively extended by the ears with the hands together or apart; the gaze is forward or up to the fingertips.

9. WARRIOR 1 WITH BREATH MOVEMENT—VIRABHADRASANA A WITH MOVEMENT

See page 119 for visual cues from the Fighting Warrior sequence.

Start in Warrior 1, bring arms to relax alongside the body, lift arms up over the head, exhale, bend at the elbows drawing the shoulder blades down the back, inhale moving into a gentle upper backbend, exhale, return to starting position, and repeat 5 to 10 times.

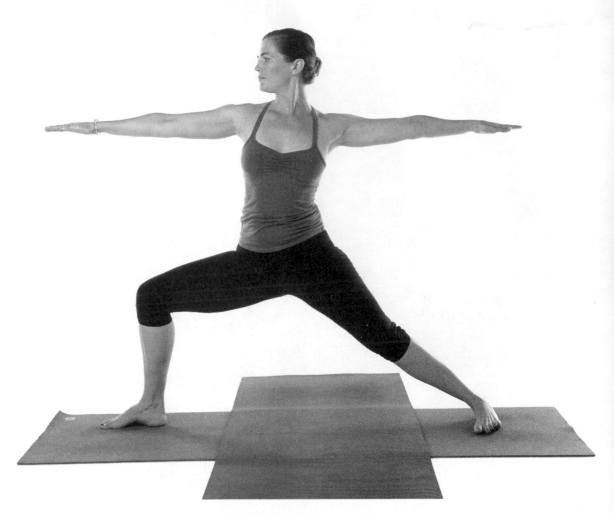

10. WARRIOR 2—VIRABHADRASANA B

Feet are at a minimum 3 feet apart with the leading foot at 90 degrees and the back foot at a 45-degree angle, hips are open and the leading leg is bent so that the thigh is parallel to the ground and the ankle and knee are in alignment, back leg is straight, torso is upright with an active spine, arms are extended out strong parallel to the ground and in alignment with the shoulders, the gaze is over the leading shoulder to the fingertips.

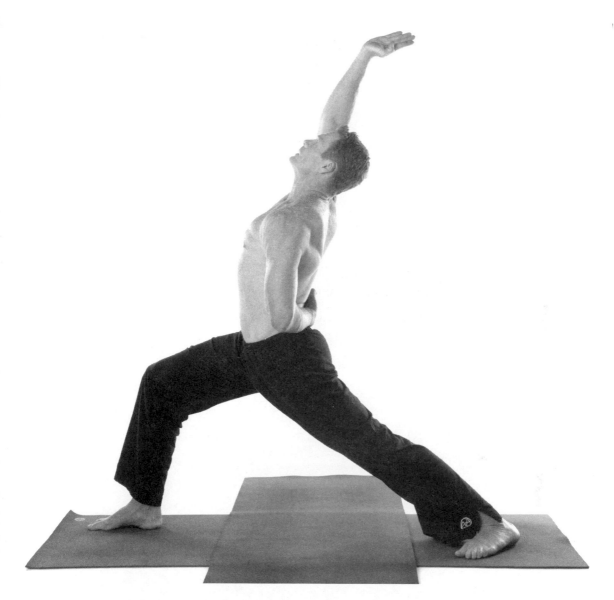

11. EXALTED WARRIOR—VIRABHADRASANA WITH BACKBEND

Start in Warrior 1. Leading hand reaches up and back as you move deep into the lunge and take an upper backbend. Opposite hand wraps around the waist and the hand is placed on the lower back or on the opposite hip.

12. DILIGENT WARRIOR—PARIVRTTA VIRABHADRASANA

See page 161 for visual cues from the Hip Mobility Drill supporting sequence.

Feet are at a minimum 3 feet apart with the leading foot at 90 degrees and the back foot at a 65-degree angle. Hips are aligned and the leading leg is bent so that the thigh is parallel to the ground, knee and ankle are in alignment, and the back leg is straight, hands are in prayer position at the heart center and the opposite elbow to the leading leg is assisting in a deep twist that starts at the base of the spine spiraling up to the top of the head, the gaze is at the tip of the nose, and the abdominals are engaged.

13. KNEELING WARRIOR 1, 2, 3—ANJANEYASANA

See page 161 for visual cues from the Hip Mobility Drill supporting sequence.

Start in high lunge, bring back leg, knee and top of foot onto the ground; arms straight by the ears leading leg knee to track past the ankle and over the toes; interlace fingers behind the back and squeeze shoulder blades, elbows, and palms toward one another, continue to lift chest and take a deeper backbend; release the hands coming out of the backbend as you bend the back leg, take the same hand as back leg and grab the outside of the ankle or foot bringing the heel to the hip (this stretches the quadriceps), opposite hand rests lightly on leading thigh.

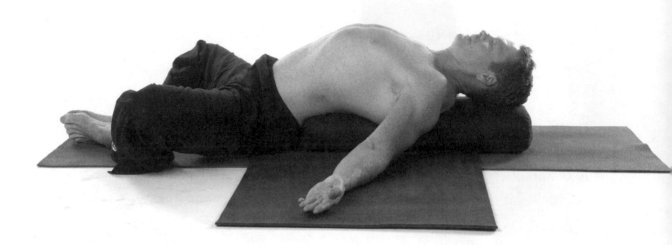

14. RESTING WARRIOR—SUPTA BADDHA KONASANA

Start in Butterfly 1. With a bolster or rolled-up blankets parallel to the spine, gently lean back so that you are supported by the props and can completely relax, palms face up, eyes closed.

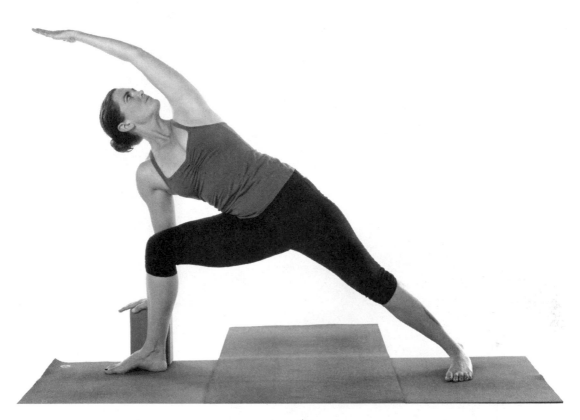

15. STANDING SIDE ANGLE POSE—UTTHITA PARSVAKONASANA

Starting in Warrior 2 reach out with your leading hand and either rest your elbow on the bent thigh or place your hand on the outside of your foot, extend your other arm at an angle in alignment with your back leg with your palm facing the floor and the fingers together. Gaze up toward your palm or elbow.

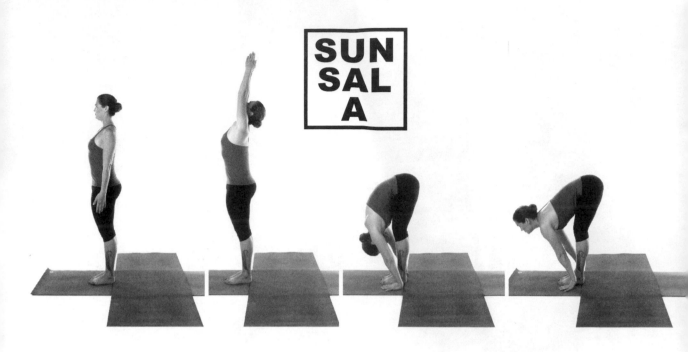

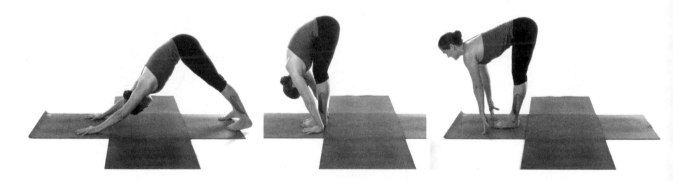

16. SUN SALUTATION A—SURYA NAMASKARA A

Start in Mountain Pose. Inhale, arms over the head, and look up. Exhale, Forward Fold, inhale, extend the back and look forward. Exhale, plant your hands on the floor, and step or jump back into plank and continue into a push-up. Inhale, Up Dog, exhale, Downward Dog (take 5 breaths

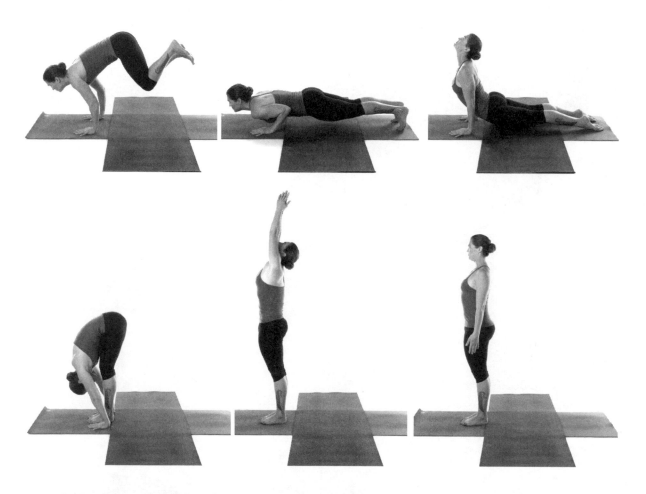

in Downward Dog). After your last exhale, look forward and walk or jump to the top of your mat, inhale, extend back, and look forward. Exhale, Forward Fold, inhale, strong legs arms out and around as you come back to standing bringing arms over the head. Exhale, back to Mountain Pose.

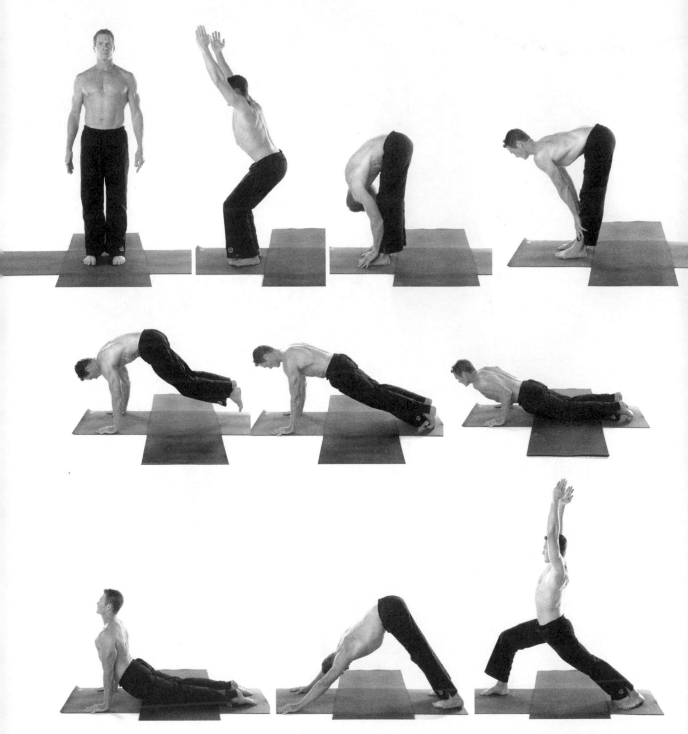

REPEAT ON LEFT SIDE AFTER VINYASA

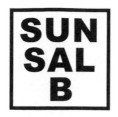

17. SUN SALUTATION B—SURYA NAMASKARA B

Standing in Mountain Pose, inhale, arms over the head, and look up as you sit into Chair Pose. Exhale, Forward Fold, inhale, extend the back, and look forward. Exhale, plant your hands, and step or jump back into plank and continue into a push-up. Inhale, Up Dog, exhale, Downward Dog, inhale, step your right foot forward, and land in Warrior 1 and hold the pose for 3 breaths. On exhale bring hands to the ground, step back, and go through a push-up. Inhale to Up Dog, exhale, Downward Dog, inhale, step the left foot forward into Warrior 1 and hold the pose 3 breaths. On exhale bring hands to the ground, step back, and go through a push-up. Inhale to Up Dog, exhale, Downward Dog, and hold the pose for 5 breaths. After your last exhale, look forward and walk or jump to the top of your mat, inhale, extend back, and look forward. Exhale, Forward Fold, inhale, strong legs arms out and around as you come back to Chair. Exhale, back to Mountain Pose.

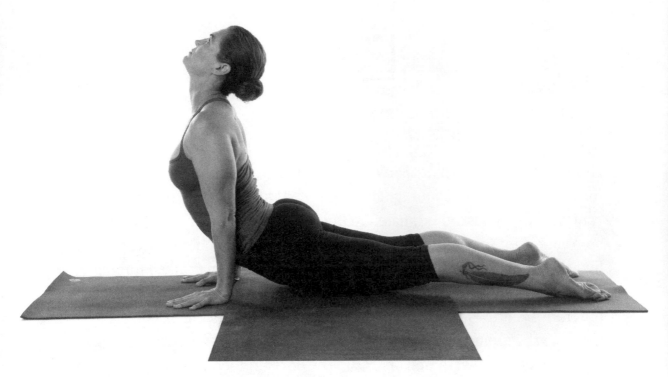

18. UPWARD-FACING DOG—URDHVA MUKHA SVANASANA

Hands are under the shoulders or slightly back and the hips and thighs are lifted as you press the tops of your feet into the ground. Your gaze is upward with a long neck as you take an upper backbend.

19. COBRA POSE—BHUJANGASANA

See page 78 for visual cues from the Zen Warrior sequence.

Hands are alongside the upper rib cage or under the shoulders and the thighs are on the ground. You are still pressing into the tops of the feet as you lift only the chest off the ground in a gentle backbend.

20. CHAIR POSE—UTKATASANA

See page 198 for visual cues from the Sun Salutation B sequence.

Feet are either together or hip-width apart. Hips, knees, and ankles are all in alignment, active spine, and the weight is slightly in the heels of the feet so that you can see all 10 toes, the arms are straight by the ears, and the gaze is upward.

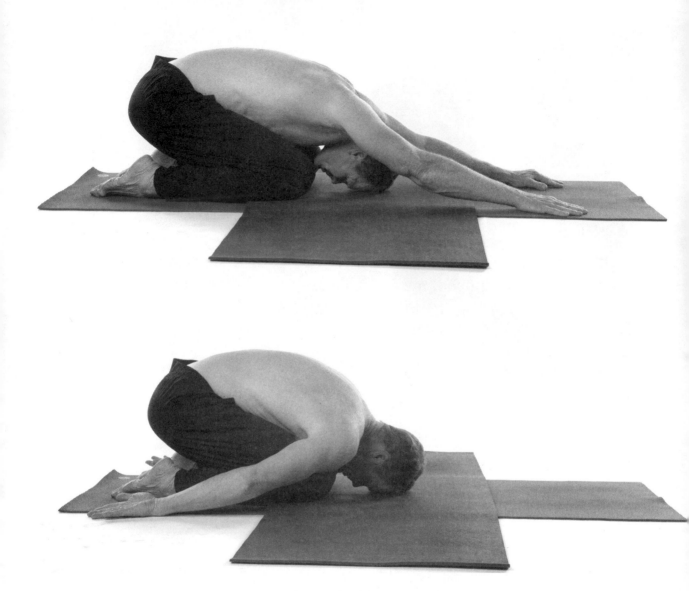

21. GRATEFUL WARRIOR—BALASANA

Bring your knees wide apart, rest your forehead on the floor or a block, arms are stretched out in front of you or alongside the body. This pose is a posture of relaxation and surrender.

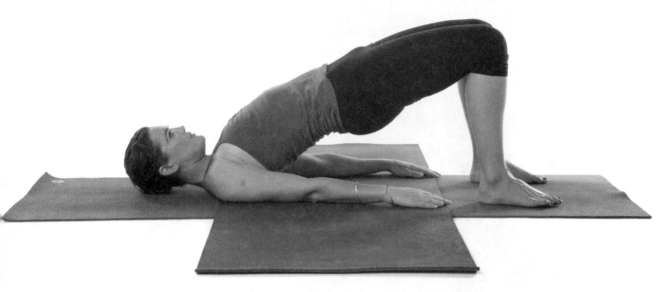

22. BRIDGE POSE—SETU BANDHA SARVANGASANA

Lying flat on the back with knees bent, feet hip-width apart, arms alongside the body, palms are facing the ground, feet firmly planted, and the knees in alignment with the heels, press into the ground with palms, shoulders, and feet. Lift hips to the sky while engaging the inner-thigh muscles. Arms and hands can remain in their initial position or if you need more support, bring hands to the lower back and elbows onto the floor.

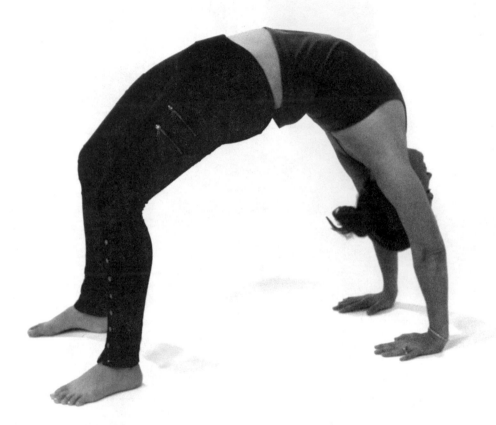

23. WHEEL POSE—CHAKRASANA OR URDHVA DHANURASANA

Lying flat on the back with knees bent and hands under the shoulders with fingertips facing the heels, elbows are pointed to the ceiling, at the same time press palms and feet into the ground to lift the body into a backbend as the shoulder blades draw toward one another and away from the ears, and the inner thighs and hamstrings engage.

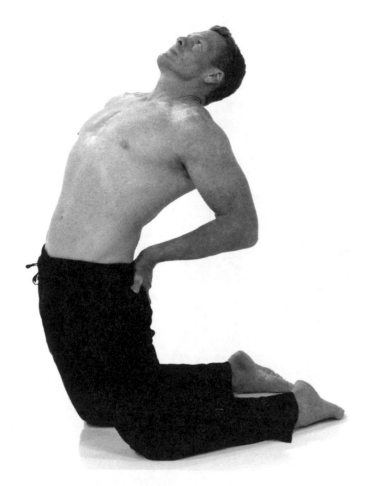

24. CAMEL POSE—USTRASANA

Standing on your knees with the toes tucked under, hips, knees, and ankles are all aligned, and hamstrings are engaged. Hands are as if you were putting your fingertips in your back pockets, rotating the inner thighs toward one another. Imagine your body creating the shape of a rainbow and begin and maintain the arch from the upper back as you move into the backbend.

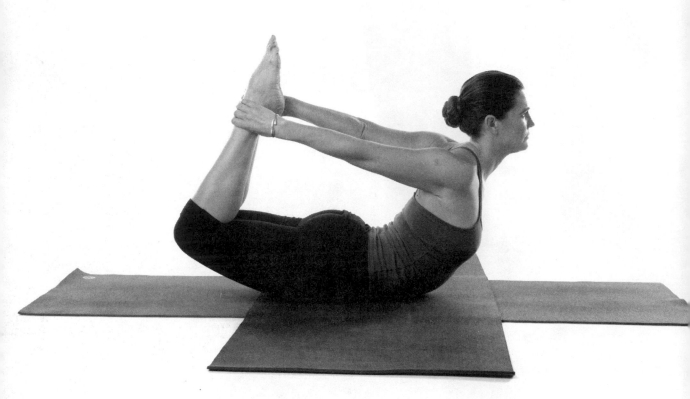

25. BOW—DHANURASANA

Lying on your belly, bend your knees, and hold on to the outside of your ankles with the thumbs pointing down. Bring feet together or at hip-width apart, keep knees at hip-width apart, press belly and hips into the ground, and lift feet toward the ceiling. Inner thighs and hamstrings are engaged as well as the back muscles, reach the chest forward, and gaze softly up.

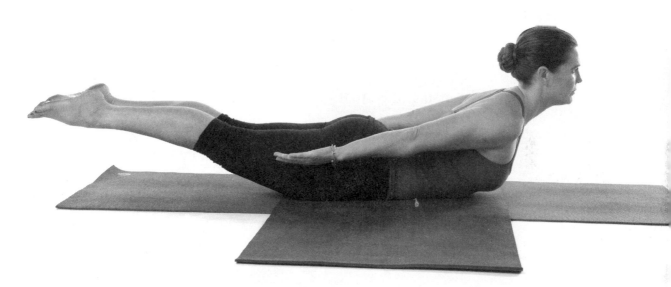

26. LOCUST—SALABHASANA

This backbend starts lying on your belly, legs straight, and big toes together. Back of the hands are on the ground alongside the hips, press into the ground with belly, hands, and hips, as you use the posterior chain to lift the body.

27. BACK ALIGNMENT—APANASANA (WITH OR WITHOUT MOVEMENT)

Lying on the back with the knees drawn into the chest, hands are on the knees and the arms are straight, inhale, exhale, use abdominals to press your sacrum into the ground as you bend the elbows and hug the knees close to the chest, inhale, return to start position, repeat 5 to 10 times, without movement; bend elbows and hug knees into chest.

28. CLEANSING WARRIOR—EKA PADA APANASANA

See page 56 for visual cues from the Peaceful Warrior sequence.

Lying on the back with the knees drawn into the chest, straighten the left leg to the ground so that the heel is on the ground and both feet are still flexed, take both hands below the right knee on the shin and bend elbows engaging the biceps and triceps, switch to the other side.

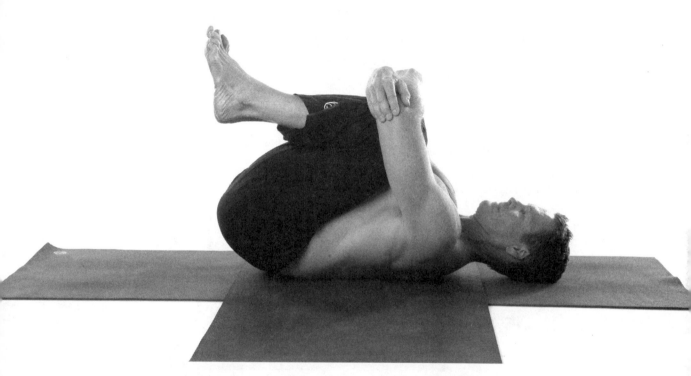

29. HEALTHY WARRIOR—SUPTA MATSYENDRASANA

Lying on the back with both knees drawn into the chest, take the hands to the knees, and draw the knees into the body. Engage abdominals as you twist extending arms out like the letter T.

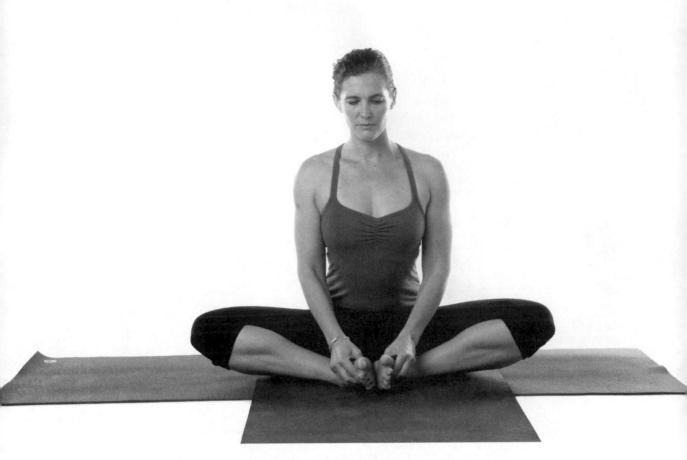

30. BUTTERFLY 1—BADDHA KONASANA 1

Sitting with feet together and knees bent, take your hands to the outside of the feet and open them up so that the pinky toes are touching and the big toes are moving outward toward the ground, knees are actively moving toward the floor, abdominals engaged, chin to chest.

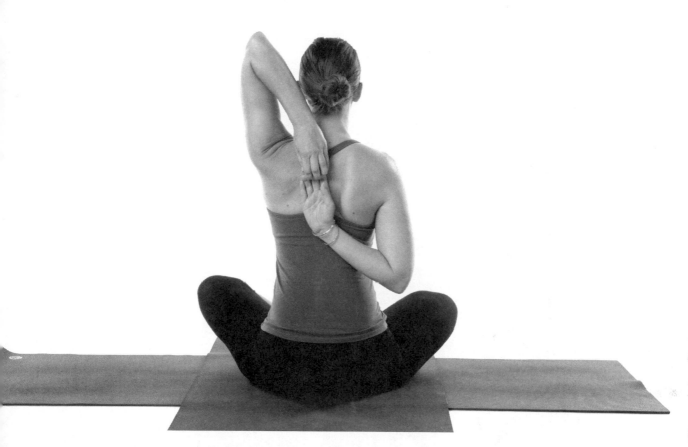

31. SHOULDER OPENER—BADDHA KONASANA WITH GOMUKHASANA ARMS

Sit in Butterfly 1, inhale, bring arms out to the side, stretch up 1 arm alongside the head, lower the other arm as it externally rotates, and you bring that hand between the shoulder blades, bend the lifted arm and meet the hands interlacing the fingers. If this pose is unachievable, grab a strap as a prop for assistance.

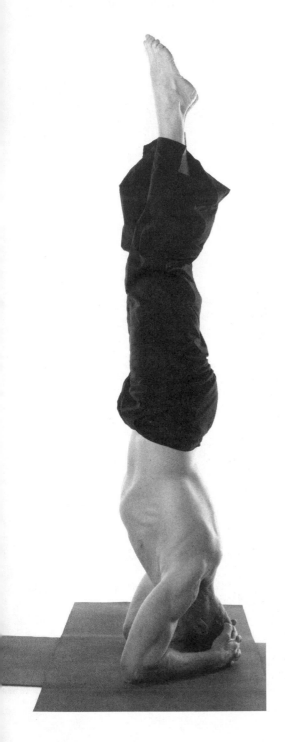

32. HEADSTAND—SIRSASANA

Begin with knees on the ground and create a base by bringing the hands, interlaced wrists, and elbows on the ground in a triangle shape. Palms create a cup for the back of your head as you place the top of your head on the ground, shift legs into a Downward Dog position, walk the legs in toward the body, lift legs into the air using core strength. No weight on the head, action is in the arms and core.

33. SHOULDER STAND— SARVANGASANA

Start lying flat on your back with arms over your head, inhale, exhale, bring your legs behind you as you bring the arms along the side of the body, toes meet the floor behind you, the legs are very active, the neck still has its natural curve, and the weight is in the shoulders. Place palms on lower back, inhale, bring the legs over the head in alignment with the hips, feet are pointed.

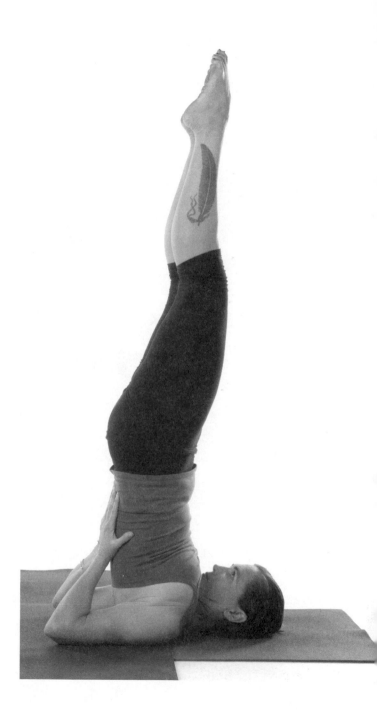

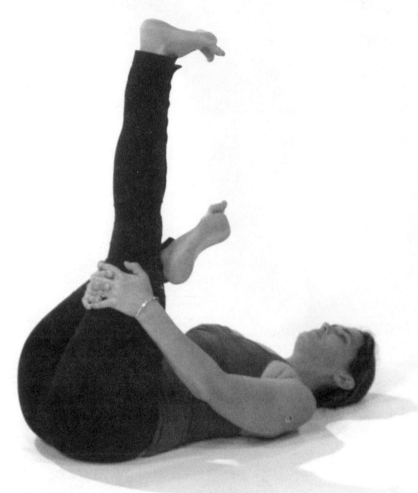

34. RECLINED PIGEON—VARIATION ON BACK OF SUPTA RAJAKAPOTASANA

Lying on the back with knees bent and feet on the ground at hip width, take the right ankle to the opposite knee, feet are flexed, thread right arm through the thighs, and interlace the fingers at the back of the left thigh, draw the left knee into chest (leg can remain bent or straightened), continue to draw the right knee away from the body and left knee toward the body.

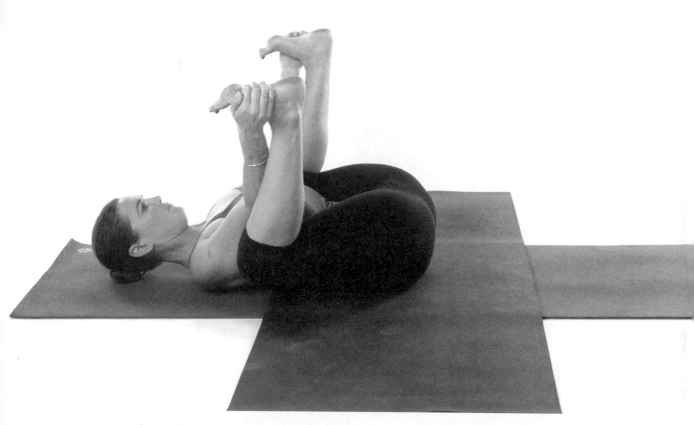

35. HAPPY BABY POSE—BALASANA

Lying on your back, bring knees into the chest and then straighten the legs up so that the feet are facing ceiling, separate legs a bit wider than hip-width apart, bend the knees taking hands to the back of the thighs, calves, ankles, or feet. Bring knees to the outside of the rib cage as you actively press feet toward the sky while pulling down with your hands.

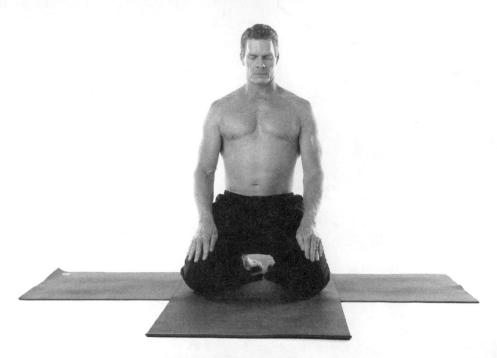

36. SEATED MEDITATION—SUKHASANA

Sitting on a chair, bench, pillow, block, blanket, or the ground, make sure you are comfortable, and your abdominals and spine are active. Top of the head is like an antenna open and receptive, abdominals are engaged, and the palms rest on the thighs or knees facing up or down.

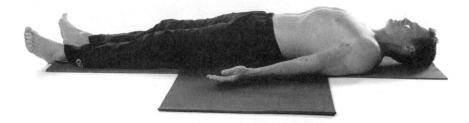

37. RESTING "DEAD MAN" POSE—SAVASANA

This pose is where you let go completely and allow yourself to be present and still. You are lying flat on your back with your arms relaxed by your sides, palms facing up, and feet relaxed. This pose is a practice of nonattachment and release. Practice breathing without effort; surrender yourself into your breathing.

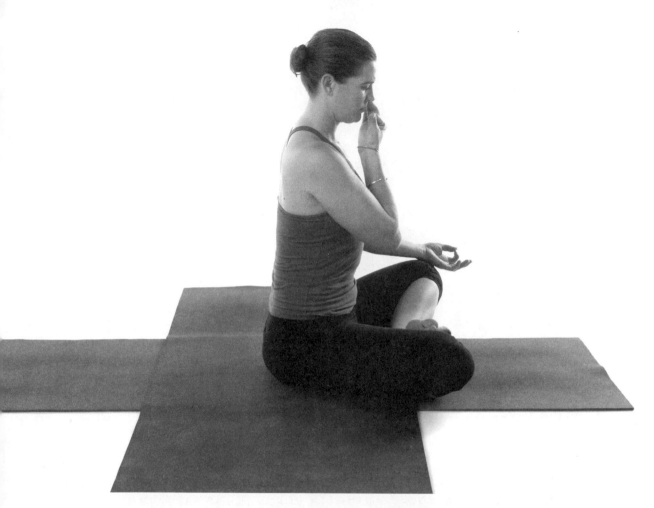

38. ALTERNATE NOSTRIL BREATHING—NADI SHODHANA

Sit in a comfortable position with the spine active and abdominals engaged. Left palm is resting on the left knee; right hand has the middle and pointer finger tucked in so that the ring, pinky, and thumb are all extended. To start, exhale the air out completely, close the right nostril lightly with the thumb, and inhale through the left. Close both nostrils using the thumb and the ring finger and hold the breath. Keeping the left nostril closed, exhale through the right. You can do this sequence with or without retentions.

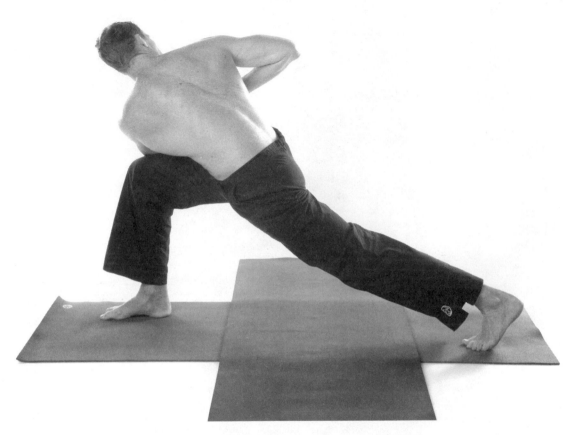

39. TWISTING WARRIOR—PARIVRTTA PARSVAKONASANA VARIATION

Start in Warrior 1. Shift back foot so that you are on the ball of the foot and pressing out through the heel in a lunge. Inhale, exhale, move hands to prayer position at the heart center, engage the abdominals as you hook opposite elbow to leading leg, twist from the base of the spine through the top of the head, eyes gazing gently over the shoulder, engage the legs, stay strong in your lines of energy.

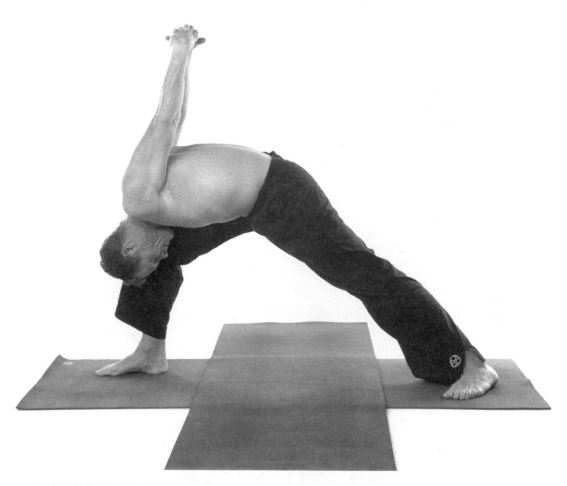

40. HUMBLE WARRIOR

Feet are about 2.5 to 3 feet apart with the leading foot at a 90 degree angle and the back foot at a 65 degree angle. Hips are squared and the leading leg is bent so that the thigh is parallel to the ground and the back leg is straight. Arms are behind with the fingers interlocked while squeezing the shoulders together. The warrior is bowing forward so that the leading shoulder is on the inside of the leading leg and the chin is sealed to the chest. The gaze is at the nose.

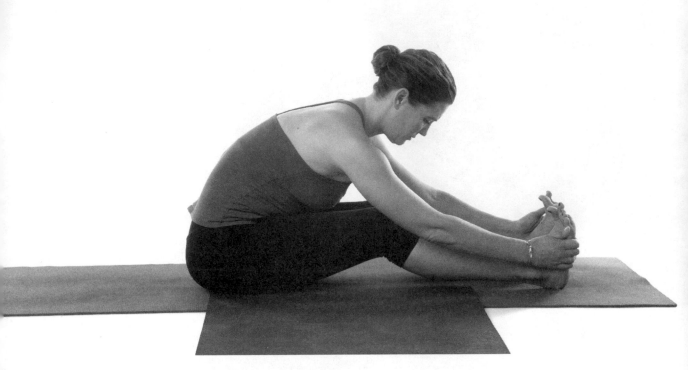

41. SEATED FORWARD FOLD—PASCHIMOTTANASANA

Sitting strong with legs out in front, feet are active, inhale, reach arms above the head, exhale, Forward Fold placing hands or a strap around the feet, keep drawing the belly button toward the spine as you press out through the balls and heels of your feet.

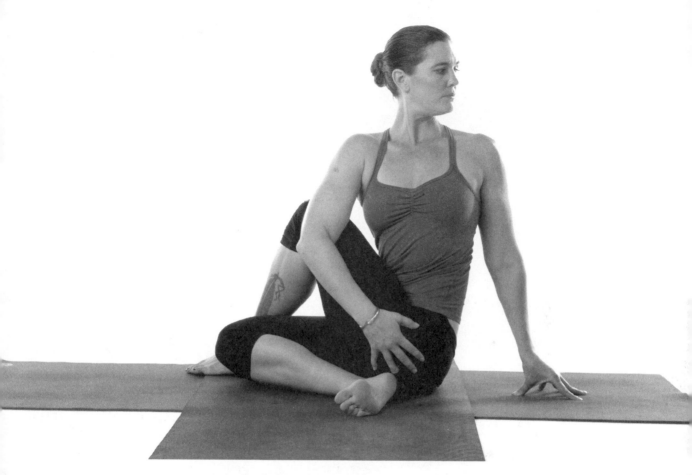

42. WISE WARRIOR 1—MARICHYASANA

Sitting upright, start with folding left leg so that the heel is alongside the right hip. Bring the right foot to the outside of the left thigh, right knee facing the ceiling, place your right hand behind you. Inhale, left arm up, exhale. Engaged in the abdominal twist, bring your left elbow or hand to the outside of your right knee, top of the head parallel to the ceiling, and both sit bones on the ground. Wise Warrior 1 variation— with the bottom leg straight.

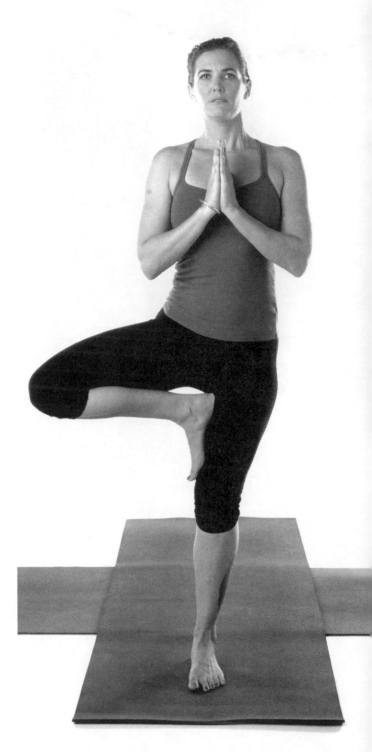

43. TREE POSE—VRKSASANA

Start in Mountain Pose. Shift weight onto left leg and lift the right leg up. Take the lifted leg's foot to the inside of the standing leg's calf or thigh. Do not put the foot on the knee joint, press the leg into the foot and the foot into the leg. Hands are in prayer position at the front of the chest.

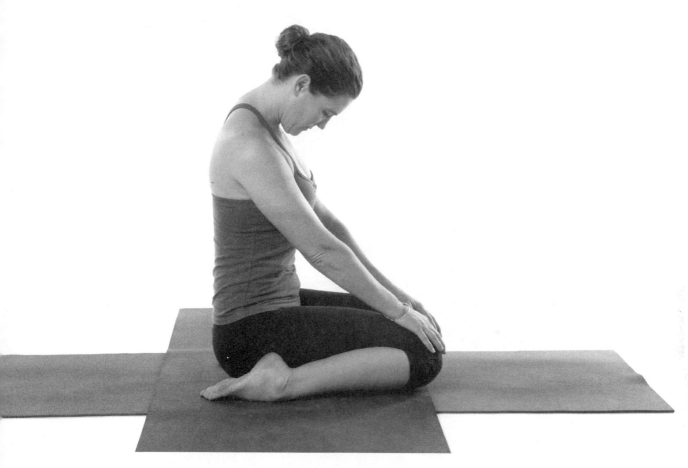

44. VICTORIOUS WARRIOR—VIRASANA

Start on your knees, bring the knees together or at hip-width apart, and sit on the inside of your feet so that the heels touch your hips. Press the tops of your feet into the ground and rotate your inner thighs toward one another, knees are touching the ground (if they are not, sit on a block), hands are on the knees, and the chin is on the chest. Gaze is at the tip of the nose.

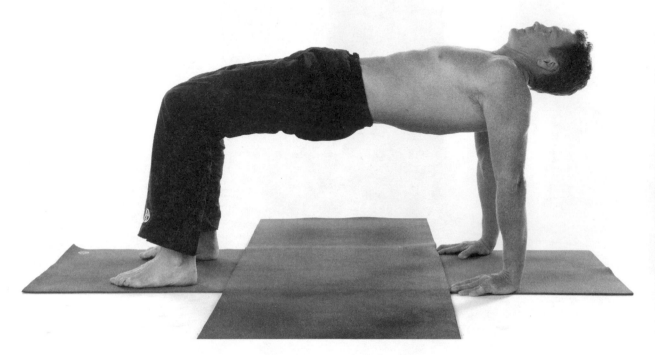

45. TABLETOP—PURVOTTANASANA VARIATION

Start lying on your back, bring feet to the ground, knees and ankles in alignment, bring hands under the shoulders with palms on the floor, press into the hands and the feet as you lift your body up, engage the posterior chain, gaze at the tip of the nose.

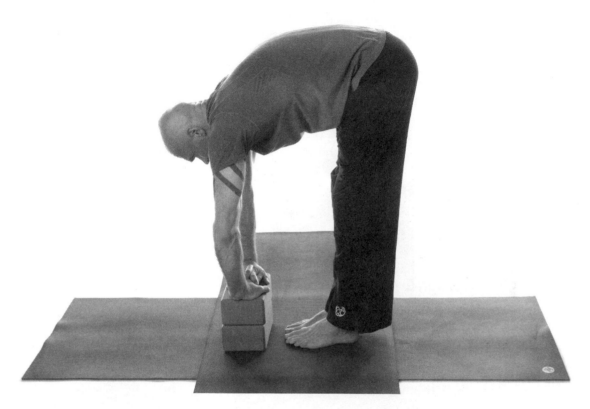

46. QIGONG, OR WATER MILL WITH FORWARD FOLD

Use blocks if necessary. Looks like Forward Fold, but it so much more.

Main components:

Weight on balls of feet

Legs pressing together, ankles, calves, knees, thighs

Fingers clasped, hands pressing into blocks

Breathing deep to lower Dantian

Active through pose

Inhale, remember to press legs, exhale, press down with hands

Exit roll spine up

Press down with hands, keep pressing legs

47. BRINGING DOWN THE HEAVENS

See page 62 for visual cues from the Peaceful Warrior sequence.

Bend the knees. Inhale and with very soft muscles arc the hands out to each side, out and then up to the face with palms slightly turned toward the body, exhale and lower hands down the midline. The intention is to be completely relaxed and balance the energies of Sky/Heaven and Earth/Yin Yang. On the inhale, imagine collecting earth energy and when the hands reach the level of the shoulders, imagine taking in the energy of the sky. On the exhale intend to balance those energies in the your body. Pose is also done to help wipe the slate clean exercise.

STANDING QIGONG MEDITATION

Knees are bent slightly, weight on the front 1/3 of your feet. Hips are tucked gently. Lengthen spine up from the base to the top of your head. Soften all the muscles and pay attention to the space that your body occupies. Breath is slow and deep to the lower abdomen.

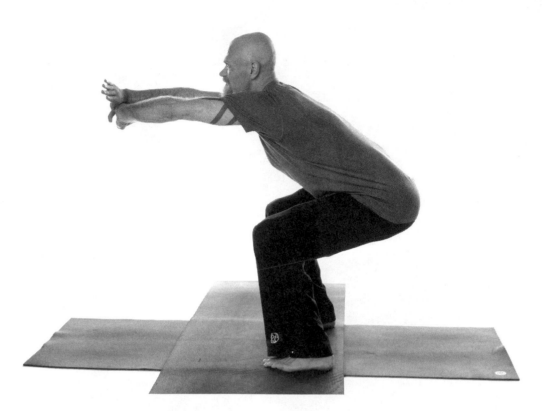

48. NARROW HORSE STANCE

Feet are shoulders width and toes are very slightly pointing in. Knees bent to 90 degrees or as close as you can get. Arms are actively pressing out in front, right hand over left. Shoulders are actively pressing down. Eyes are focused straight ahead looking at the back of your hands. Knees should be active pressing in like you are trying to hold a medicine ball between them. Keep your spine as straight as possible. This is a survival exercise, so do your best to maintain form for 3 minutes: It will be challenging. To finish, turn palms into fists, rise up on your toes while bringing your fists into you ben elbows; pulling your hands in and drawing the energy. Then step your feet together, turn palms down, and press down with both hands holding them with fingertips facing forward, wrists extended. Press the legs together as in the Water Mill—extended forward bend. Take 3 deep breaths while continuing to press the legs together.

49. DANCING WARRIOR— NATARAJASANA

Standing with feet together, shift weight to the left foot and lift right foot toward your buttocks. Take your right hand and grab the inside or outside of your right foot. Bring the left arm straight by your head and begin to kick your right foot into your right hand as you reach your chest forward and create an arch with the back: 50 percent back, 50 percent forward.

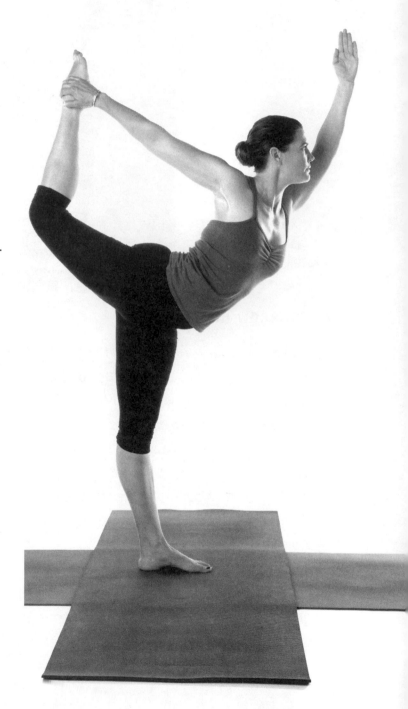

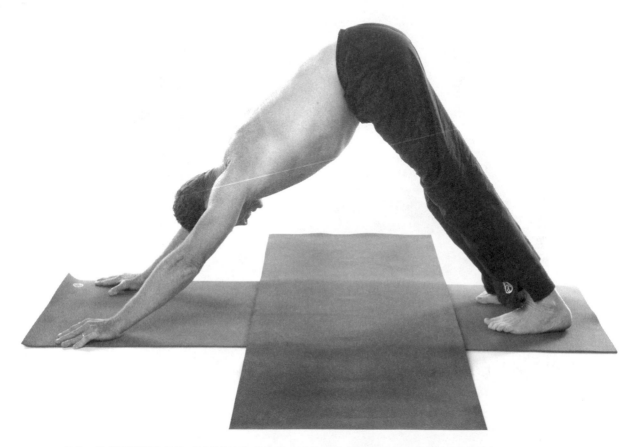

50. DOWNWARD-FACING DOG—ADHO MUKHA SVANASANA

With your hands and feet on the ground your body is creating an inverted-V position. Quadriceps are engaged and your heels are on the ground or moving in that direction. All knuckles of your hands are pressing into the ground as you engage your abdominals and lift your sit bones toward the ceiling.

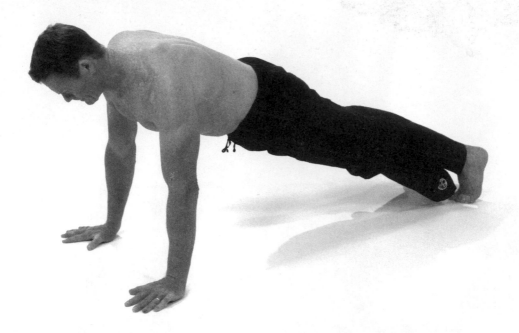

51. PLANK

Strong, stafflike position with the whole body. Hands are pressing firmly into the ground. It is like the beginning of a push-up. Press the heels toward the wall behind you as you balance on your toes. Whole body is engaged.

52. WARRIOR BREATH

Warrior Breath is a strong inhale and exhale through the nose to the upper chest. The focus is on the inhale. Slightly rock your upper body back as you inhale. Slightly rock forward with the exhale. The most important component to remember is that it is a warrior's breath, so it is strong. Take 9 (or more breaths for each set). On the last breath hold for 3 seconds, swallow down, and round out your abdomen. Keep abdomen gently pressing out as you exhale slowly through your lips. The exhale is called the Eternal Exhale. Some people take 2 to 3 minutes to exhale completely. During this exhale relax and visualize.

CHAPTER 7

PHYSIOLOGICAL AND PSYCHOLOGICAL BENEFITS OF YOGA

Yoga is not a religion. It is science, science of well-being, science of youthfulness, science of integrating body, mind and soul.
—AMIT RAY

IN THIS CHAPTER WE WILL TAKE A LOOK AT CURRENT RESEARCH ON THE MANY BENEFITS OF YOGA, AND KOKORO YOGA IN PARTICULAR. BUT BEFORE WE DIG THROUGH SOME OF THE MODERN RESEARCH THAT HAS EMERGED IN RECENT YEARS THAT HAS HELPED SCIENTISTS UNDERSTAND WHAT A YOGA PRACTICE CAN DELIVER, I FIRST WANT TO ENCOURAGE YOU TO BE YOUR OWN SCIENTIST: TO HONOR ANY SKEPTICISM YOU MAY HAVE AND FIND A BALANCED APPROACH to being analytical in your appraisal of yoga, but to also be rigorous and dedicated to testing it out for yourself.

I'm a big believer in trusting through verification. By giving this training a concentrated, objective, personal trial, you'll be able to verify the benefits I'm discussing. What I don't want to see you do is to slide into the trap of prejudging yoga as an excuse to not give it a valid try.

Lack of time also should not be a barrier. Kokoro Yoga is designed for a busy individual going 100 mph, and I wouldn't have it any other way. So even if it's 5 or 10 minutes a day for 3 months, I encourage you to conduct your own science by testing out the program and noting how it works for you.

Yoga has thousands of years of subjective science within its foundation, but for the Western audience seeking validation from a peer-reviewed research study, it's only in recent years that we have plowed deeper into the subject. Scientists and medical professionals—in pursuit of effective, low-cost health-care solutions, are using high-tech tools to uncover the most detailed and objective data in history. For example, they are now able to chart changes in brain growth and function (neoplasticity), hormonal and electrical patterns associated with thoughts and emotions, and changes in gene expressions from exercise that lead to physiological improvements (epigenetics). There's much about yoga that I believe is still out of the current range of modern science to test, but I'm confident that if you integrate Kokoro Yoga rituals and disciplines into your life, you won't care about what the scientists say, you will just love the benefits and growth you are experiencing.

BENEFITS ACROSS THE SPECTRUM

The following is a holistic review of the benefits, both physiological and psychological, of what you can expect to get from a disciplined, daily practice:

Body Control

Yoga develops body control through an acute awareness of body position and movement. This control extends to awareness of how you move safely and effectively throughout each day: from standing to walking, running, lifting, or even the inherently unhealthy act of sitting. It will allow you to maintain connection with and move from your center (the Hara in Japanese and Dantian in Chinese), and extend to control over your physiological adaptation to stress.

Core Strength

As mentioned earlier, yoga shares a common history with the martial arts, and engaging the core of your body while moving is a focus of the movement practice. If you have some training in martial arts, then you know what I mean by this. Others will have to experience it. You will learn to sink into a stable position of deep balance and engage all the muscles of your core as your primary source of physical strength and stability. Too often we focus on the extremities (arms and legs) in training, ignoring the critical source of power of the core, which is more than one's abs. It is the entire body minus the limbs and head. Building a strong core starts with deep connection to the muscles protecting the spine, engaging the root near your tailbone, and extending to all of the supporting muscles of your glutes, lower back, abs, chest, and obliques.

Concentration

In yoga practice, you sharpen your ability to concentrate on one thing, and for long periods of time, by focusing your mind on a single point, such as your breathing or the structure of a pose. Research clearly supports how this brand of exercise elevates the ability to concentrate. In one study, 60 subjects were involved in a 3-month retreat where they practiced focusing on the breath. The group was split into those who participated in the practice and those who were on a wait-list group that weren't. The test they were given involved watching lines flash on a computer screen. Each time they saw a line that they believed was shorter than the others, their job was to click the mouse, an exceptionally boring task where the mind was apt to wander. Those performing concentration practice consistently demonstrated significantly greater capacity to focus than those who weren't. As reported when the study was published in 2010, the researchers at University of California, Davis, wrote, "Training produced improvements in visual discrimination that were linked to increases in perceptual sensitivity and improved vigilance during sustained visual attention."

Flexibility and Durability

For many, this is the sum total of what yoga is expected to deliver. Through the work of the sequences, you develop flexibility of your muscles and durability of your spine, joints, and connective tissues.

Energy Integrity

Controlling and enhancing energy, which can be conceptualized as life force, through breath control and visualization drills. Learning to draw energy into the body, to move it, and enliven the body at a cellular level, comes from a long-term practice of yoga.

Detoxification

One of the first benefits I registered in my initial exposure to Hot Yoga was the detoxification of the muscles, the blood, and the organs. We accomplish this in Kokoro Yoga without the need for a superheated room by using breathing techniques and, of course, vigorous movement. These detox benefits can be keen for desk warriors in the world. Prolonged sitting not only degrades the tissues of the hip capsule, but also weakens and shortens all of the machinery of the trunk that protects the spine. As you can feel after unhinging yourself from the window seat after a long flight, prolonged periods of sitting shut off the lymphatic system and retard the removal of waste products from the muscles, connective tissues, and nervous system.

Improved Immune Function

Hard-charging athletes typically have some experience in what is often referred to as "over-training syndrome." Overtraining means, obviously, the athlete has been overdoing it: relentless training without adequate recovery. Symptoms include chronic fatigue, iron deficiency, states of depression, upper-respiratory infections, and a sharp decline in performance. This syndrome is not limited to the sports arena: special operators, first responders, and those in high-stress business pursuits can also get caught in this psychophysical quicksand. When decline in performance begins to show up in the training journal, the highly motivated individual can react by training even harder, making things worse.

In specific regard to overtraining and the prevention of overtraining, first consider the vast complexity of the immune system, with multilayers of protection throughout the body that works tirelessly to screen out or kill viruses, microbes, pathogens, and cancers.

As you'll note from the chart, the quality of your immune function is affected not just by training but by just about every part of your life that you can imagine. Stress is stress,

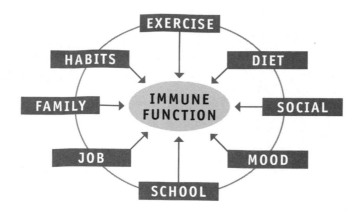

and if on top of your training stress, you are absorbing vast amounts of stress, incurred from either bad diet, lack of sleep, poor relationships, and the like, then your immune system will ultimately fall into what is known as immunosuppression.

Along with the basic habits of good health, like a smart diet, drinking plenty of water, and getting adequate sleep, consistent yoga practice will help boost your immune function. A 2013 Bloomberg article reported that, "Scientists are getting close to proving what yogis have held to be true for centuries—yoga and meditation can ward off stress and disease." The story centered on a 5-year study being conducted at the Harvard Medical School that was examining the effects of yoga and meditation on brain activity and gene function.

John Denninger, a psychiatrist at Harvard Medical School, is leading the study on how the practices affect genes and brain activity in the chronically stressed. His latest work follows a study he and others published earlier this year showing how so-called mind-body techniques can switch on and off some genes linked to stress and immune function. Using neuroimaging and genomics technologies, Denninger and his colleagues are finding that yoga can switch specific genes, related to immune function, on and off, and how yoga can play a powerful role in reducing hypertension and preventing depression. "There is a true biological effect," he told Bloomberg. "The kinds of things that happen when you meditate do have effects throughout the body, not just in the brain."

In another key study conducted at Ohio State, surgical nurses, who experienced high levels of stress through their work and proximity to death, were shown to have a 40 percent decrease in salivary alpha amylase, a stress marker, after practicing yoga on a consistent basis.

Longevity

Neuroscientists have come to believe that the toll of aging on the human body and brain is an outcome of disuse rather than use. In fact, in pioneering research conducted in the 1970s at the University of California (Berkeley and San Francisco), it was discovered that the brain responds favorably, at the microscopic level, to movement and stimulating experience. It was when usage came to a stop that the part of the brain associated with the usage weakened.

In this study, the scientists determined that the brain was "neuroplastic," a term meant to describe how connections between brain cells are circuitlike—strengthening, changing, or weakening in response to how and how much the circuits are being used.

The implications of the neuroplasticity model are huge. In a long-term study performed at Cardiff University in the United Kingdom, researchers took a detailed look at the effects of exercise and lifestyle choices on 2,235 men, ages 45 to 49, over the course of 30 years. The results were powerful: consistent exercise was the most cogent factor in reducing the risk of dementia by 60 percent. In reporting on the magnitude of this study, *The Wall Street Journal* said, "Imagine if there were a drug that could reduce the risk of dementia by 60%. It would be the most talked-about drug in history."

Brain exercise has been shown to improve cognitive computing power against the grain of decline normally associated with aging. After completing 10 1-hour brain exercise sessions, 2 per week over the course of a month and a half, the subjects demonstrated remarkable effects on their ability to think, reason, and function even 10 years after the brain exercise workouts.

That's just the beginning when it comes to what a mental training exercise, like meditation, can do. Studies at the University of California, Davis, have looked at the effect that meditation has on telomerase activity in the brain—telomerase is known as the "immortality enzyme."

The key action can be found in the infinitesimal corners of genes in what are called "telomeres." Telomeres are found at the ends of chromosomes in sequences of DNA. Typically, they shorten every time the cell divides, and when they get too short, the cell dies. Telomerase actively rebuilds and lengthens the telomeres, consequently promoting a longer cell life, and studies have suggested that by higher amounts of telomerase equates to improved states of mental and physical health, and that it can have a direct role in preventing stress-related aging rates.

Researchers at UCLA found that a mere 12 minutes of yoga per day, increased telomerase by 43 percent.

Increased Stamina and Endurance

In a study published in 2013, researchers in Boston took a high-tech look at what they termed the "relaxation response" that occurs from yoga and meditation. Using blood samples taken before and after a meditation session, the blood was analyzed to extract gene transcription profiles. The results were powerful and all-encompassing: "Practice enhanced expression of genes associated with energy metabolism, mitochondrial function, insulin secretion and telomere maintenance, and reduced expression of genes linked to inflammatory response and stress-related pathways." The researchers found that the greatest benefits were harvested after a long-term practice, with improved energy metabolism and mitochondrial function some of the especially appealing benefits that an endurance athlete might be interested in.

Cognitive Performance

A New York Academy of Sciences review showcased the value of yoga in regards to cognition and mental performance, with researchers emphasizing that yoga may be an effective intervention for the elderly dealing with a decline in memory and other aspects of brain performance. The research team concluded: "Studies involved a wide variety of meditation techniques and reported preliminary positive effects on attention, memory, executive function, processing speed, and general cognition."

Decrease in Cellular Inflammation

Decreasing cellular inflammation is important for overall health, but also for peak performance. There have been some breakthrough studies being performed using blood testing that are answering the question of why yoga has a positive effect on cellular inflammation. Since cellular inflammation is one of the root causes of type 2 diabetes and chronic diseases like cancer (as well as Alzheimer's, which is predicted to join the diabetes epidemic), this finding is particularly forceful. In the athletic training world, a lot of attention is paid to the effect diet has on cellular inflammation. Basically, a crappy, high-carb diet (rich in processed foods and sugars) sends the body into a state of hyperglycemia, or chronic state of high-blood sugar, because of the fatigue associated with overtapping the insulin response that occurs when we eat a high-carb meal. Hyperglycemia is the precursor to diabetes and a host of related chronic diseases that you want to prevent at all costs. In addition to actively getting a handle on your diet, research shows that yoga and meditation can be a powerful anti-inflammatory. In a study published in *The Clinical Journal of Oncology,* Ohio State scientists looked at three different cytokine levels in the blood in breast cancer survivors. The cytokines analyzed were distinct proteins commonly used as markers for cellular inflammation levels. After 12 weeks of yoga practice, the subjects of the study showed a 10 to 15 percent lowering in all three cytokine markers.

Depression and PTSD

A 2008 RAND Corporation study indicated that one out of five combat troops that had returned from the wars in Iraq or Afghanistan met the criteria for PTSD. Incorporating an assortment of studies supporting that yoga is an effective management tool in regards to chronic depression and PTSD, psychiatric researchers at the Boston University School of Medicine took an in-depth look at the mechanisms involved with PTSD and has proposed that there are "far-reaching implications for the integration of yoga-based practices in the treatment of a broad array of disorders exacerbated by stress."

Lower Back Pain

In 2008, the Medical Expenditure Panel Survey collected a data set that suggested that 100 million American adults were affected by chronic pain, back pain, and arthritis. The study estimated that the health-care costs due to these maladies, when you add up the productivity costs and health-care costs, is in the range of $560 to $635 billion—*annually.* In 2011, the largest study ever conducted on the subject, published by the *Archives of Internal Medicine,* found that 12 weeks of yoga diminished symptoms and improved overall back function. As far as research goes, yoga has been highlighted as an answer to lower back pain, a problem that costs the United States billions in terms of lost productivity from the workforce.

Presence

Power is found by focusing on the right thing, right now. A quality of the peak performance flow state is to be fully in the moment. Not distracted by emotionally charged memories or the fear of what may happen in the future, but being comprehensively engaged with the present moment. Kokoro Yoga training will guide you on how to use your mind powerfully in the future and past, so that you don't need to dwell there, but can release those time-based mental constructs and stay in the here and now—and perform.

Fitness and Wellness

As discussed in this chapter, research has found that yoga is helpful in treating high-blood pressure, diabetes, back pain, sleep problems, depression, anxiety, stress, and more. But the benefits can be enhanced with more rigorous interval training. Before I began my practice of yoga, I tried to use yoga programs for my fitness needs. I soon learned that they were a poor substitute for real functional fitness, the type required of warriors and athletes. Though it has some cardio benefit, traditional yoga focuses mostly on balance, flexibility, and core strength. Because it is lacking in strength, stamina, work capacity, and durability, we introduced more intense functional fitness routines to Kokoro Yoga.

A POWERFUL FUTURE

My intent throughout this chapter was to explore the benefits and take a short dive into the science behind the principles in this book. I believe Kokoro Yoga is a Trojan horse ready to unleash a host of benefits, ultimately leading to the highest levels of performance and even consciousness itself. I know, it may sounds too good to be true, but if you stay with me and begin a daily routine that meets your practical needs, body type, and goals, then you will be planting the seeds for a powerful future.

REFERENCES

A quick note: I included this chapter as review of the more recent research that is currently being conducted in regards to yoga, and as such have included references so you can validate what's being learned.

Bhasin, M. K., J. A. Dusek, B-H Chang, M. G. Joseph, J. W. Denninger, et al. "Relaxation Response Induces Temporal Transcriptome Changes in Energy Metabolism, Insulin Secretion and Inflammatory Pathways." *PLoS ONE* vol. 8, no. 5 (2013): e62817. doi:10.1371/journal.pone.0062817.

"Does Yoga Really Do the Body Good?" American Council on Exercise, September/October 2005. www.acefitness.org/getfit/studies/YogaStudy2005.pdf.

Elwood, P., J. Galante, J. Pickering, S. Palmer, A. Bayer, et al. "Healthy Lifestyles Reduce the Incidence of Chronic Diseases and Dementia: Evidence from the Caerphilly Cohort Study." *PLoS ONE* vol. 8, no. 12 (2013): e81877. doi:10.1371/journal.pone.0081877.

Gaskin, D. J., Richard, P. "The Economic Costs of Pain in the United States." *Journal of Pain* vol. 13, no. 8 (2012): 715–24.

"Harvard Yoga Scientists Find Proof of Meditation Benefit." Bloomberg News, November 21, 2013. www.bloomberg.com/news/articles/2013-11-22/harvard-yoga-scientists-find-proof-of-meditation-benefit.

"Invisible Wounds of War. Psychological and Cognitive Injuries, Their Consequences, and Services to Assist Recovery." RAND Corporation, January 15, 2008. www.rand.org/content/dam/rand/pubs/monographs/2008/RAND_MG720.pdf.

Jacobs, T. L., Epel, E. S., Lin, J., Blackburn, E. H., Wolkowtiz, O. M., et al. "Intensive meditation training, immune cell telomerase activity, and psychological mediators." *Psychoneuroendocrinology* vol. 36, issue 5 (2011): 664–81.

Glaser, J., Bennett, J. M., Andridge, R., Peng, J., et al. "Yoga's Impact on Inflammation, Mood, and Fatigue in Breast Cancer Survivors: A Randomized Controlled Trial," *Journal of Clinical Oncology* vol. 32, (January 2014): 1040–1049.

Lavretsky, H., P. Siddarth, N. Nazarian, N. St. Cyr, D. S. Khalsa, et al. "A pilot study of yogic meditation for family dementia caregivers with depressive symptoms: Effects on mental health, cognition, and telomerase activity." *International Journal of Geriatric Psychiatry* vol. 28, no. 1 (2013): 57–65.

MacLean, K. A., Ferrer, E., Aichele, S. R. Bridwell, D. A., Zanesco, A. P., et al. "Intensive Meditation Training Improves Perceptual Discrimination and Sustained Attention." *Psychological Science* vol. 21, no. 6 (2010): 829–39.

Gothe, Neva P. "The effects of an 8-week Hatha yoga intervention on executive function in older adults." *Journals of Gerontology* 69 (2014): 1109–16.

Rosenzweig, M. R. "Aspects of the Search for Neural Mechanisms of Memory." *Annual Review of Psychology* 47 (1996): 1–32.

CHAPTER 8

DEVELOPING A PERSONAL PRACTICE

Today I will do what others won't, so tomorrow I can accomplish what others can't.

—NFL GREAT JERRY RICE

"TODAY I WILL DO WHAT OTHERS WON'T, SO TOMORROW I CAN ACCOMPLISH WHAT OTHERS CAN'T." THIS QUOTE IS WORTH REPEATING. IT'S WORTH TAPING TO YOUR MIRROR DURING YOUR FIRST MONTHS OF TRAINING. WHY? ONCE YOU'VE APPLIED THE DRUMBEAT OF CONSISTENCY WITH A SET OF KOKORO YOGA SEQUENCES AND RITUALS, AND HAVE MAINTAINED THE PROGRAM LONG ENOUGH FOR THE BENEFITS TO CATCH HOLD—AS IT BECOMES MESHED WITH YOUR daily routine in a way that you can't imagine missing out on—there will be no want or need to burn time trying to assess the next shiny thing or obsess about the latest double-blind, peer-reviewed research study on the subject on whether this works or not. The thing is: You'll see it, feel it, and know it.

Unfortunately, what typically happens when someone gets all revved up to start a personal development program is this: After drifting through a period with too much work, stress, and poor eating habits, self-loathing sets in. You feel like you hit a threshold where you just can't take it any longer so you begin to search. A provocative Facebook ad promises immediate transformation so you jump into a new program. The opening stage of any such undertaking is fraught with peril, as a move toward deep-rooted change in habits or our being is often met with a tidal wave of internal resistance. After 1 or 2 months, your initial high motivation meets with the ultimate truth that this takes work—the daily, routine type of work. You tell yourself that maybe this wasn't "it" and that you just don't have time for this stuff . . . you lose faith and once again begin to be push-pulled in a myriad of directions. The slow, steady erosion of physical, mental, and spiritual well-being continues anew. Sad story, but it doesn't have to be that way. It is time to truly upgrade yourself not just through faith, but with massive commitment.

"*Do. Or do not. There is no try,*" says Jedi Master Yoda of *Star Wars* fame, imploring Luke Skywalker, his disciple, to build personal power through daily disciplined practice. Trying is not committing. Commitment leads to courage, which gets us moving toward developing the skills and competencies for the task of fulfilling your mission and purpose. Fear is met head-on then tossed aside as confidence and momentum build.

Trying, on the other hand, immediately gives you an out—a back door to run through when things don't go as planned (which is always). Many languages have no word for "try," and now is a good time to erase it from yours. Language can be a prison for the rational mind, limiting your range of thought and action. Better to avoid words like "try," "could," "should," and "would," and adopt the attitude that once a decision is made, a redline is crossed—a line that can't be retraced. We simply must proceed with a "fire-in-the-belly" commitment and an "all-in" mind-set. *Do. Or do not.*

The SEALs say that you must "earn your Trident every day." The Trident is their symbol of commitment to excellence and they proudly wear it on their chest. Everyone in the sphere that they work recognizes and honors that symbol for the individual behind it and the ethos that they represent. "Self-mastery in service to humanity" sums it up. That is the same type of ethos you will be developing with this program, and you will need to sharpen your sword daily on the path.

The simplest way to look at sharpening the sword is through daily disciplined physical training and practice, a foundational principle of Kokoro Yoga. In opening up your mobility and spinal health, by increasing energy through powerful breathing techniques and recharging your physical capacity through functional movements, you are renewed with energy and growing confidence that becomes a self-perpetuating force. This leads to a clear mind, an open heart, and a connection to your true self, allowing a vision of the passion, purpose, and principles of your unique personal ethos to arise. Further integration accelerates you toward your goals, with positive energy radiating outward that attracts a team of warriors ready to support you in a mutually symbiotic, interconnected web destined to co-create a better world.

Yoga is the multilayered warrior development discipline I had been searching for ever since the day I left my NYC dojo to become a Navy SEAL. But as it turns out, I had to create it to find it. For thousands of years, yoga has been an open source project to develop a complete personal development program, but it has been largely hidden from view in modern times. Practicing Kokoro Yoga on a daily basis for weeks, months, and years offers you a single approach in which you sharpen the array of inner resources we're all born with across the spectrum of mind-body-spirit. When we sharpen our sword daily, everyone and every moment becomes our teacher. We open ourselves to the reality that we know little about the true nature of the universe and meaning of life, so we lower our heads, soften our gaze, and become lifelong learners.

The Japanese concept of "kokoro," denotes the spiritual aspect of our training. Kokoro represents our warrior's spirit and translates as "merge heart and mind in action." Kokoro training begins as a solitary journey without a true summit, and at every peak you successfully climb you will experience an unforeseen plateau, followed by a fresh climb. But on the mountain path you will taste previously untouchable realms of power and connect with fellow travelers. It is a journey of the soul, and one that you must make alone.

A CUSTOM PRACTICE

Your practice will be personal and change over time. Every individual coming to yoga has different needs, inspiration, mental and emotional development, moral bearing, body type, injury matrix, and level of fitness and spiritual beliefs. A personal practice is optimized when it can be customized. In fact, that is one of the unique and pleasant ways that Kokoro Yoga is different from most other forms or systems of yoga.

A huge challenge for us is that our lives are frenetic; racing to the yoga studio to catch a class 5 times a week can exacerbate the problem into a rolling boil. So why not train in your own bedroom, or on the beach, or in the woods? Let's customize our training so we can build "stick-to-it habits" that discipline ourselves to train daily. Let me share how Catherine and I customize our personal practices so you can get a sense of where to go with yours.

Recall that Catherine is training the Peaceful Warrior within her—so she can spread love through her teaching and personal practice. Catherine organizes her personal practice to support that archetype, and it includes a weekly dose of 2 to 3 Ashtanga group classes in the primary and secondary series and teaching 3 restorative Peaceful Warrior classes. It is supplemented with daily meditation and spot drills. She supports it with a functional fitness routine of 3 CrossFit classes and 1 to 2 moderate walks or runs. All of this is woven into her weekly schedule as it ebbs and flows. She allows for flexibility to add or subtract based on her work and travel schedule.

My personal practice is based on my warrior ethos. I practice a short morning and evening ritual and do spot drills daily (box breathing and visualization drills) to ensure that I cover all Five Mountains in my practice. I teach Kokoro Yoga at SEALFIT HQ once a week, focusing on the Fighting or Fit Warrior sequences. The meat and potatoes of my training are 2-3 moderate to long sessions and 3–4 SEALFIT WODS and 1 self-defense class where I integrate mental, emotional, and awareness skills into the training. I train for roughly 3 hours a day all told, and allow for flexibility to be spontaneous, jump into training with my team, or take a rest day. I also strive to challenge myself with something new and different every month that will test my limits.

Of course you will design your personal practice based on your intuitive sense of where you need to develop skills and close weakness gaps. Your personal practice must sync both with your warrior spirit and your lifestyle. That is the beauty of this practice—it is uniquely designed to mold to your personality and intuitively felt needs.

RITUALS, SPOT DRILLS, AND RETREATS

As I have made abundantly clear, committing to, and sticking to, a personal practice requires the development of new habits. Habits must become ritualistic for them to sink in. It may seem overwhelming to add one more thing to your schedule now . . . but don't despair! Kokoro Yoga has three key training methods that ensure your personal practice will become a discipline and then a habit. They are: 1) rituals, 2) spot drills, and 3) retreats.

The ritual is a practice session that you do every day at the same time to provide a foundation for excellence during the day. We have the morning ritual and the evening ritual. Both are integrated training sessions, seeping with power, providing important bookends to your day. If you do no other training besides these two rituals, you are good to go. I will describe the morning ritual first, followed by the evening ritual.

The Morning Ritual

It is common to wake up, grab your smartphone to check e-mails while preparing your coffee, and allow your mind and emotions to spin up. The more uncommon, Kokoro Yoga approach, is to commit to win in your mind before you step foot onto the day's battlefield. The morning ritual is an integrated session that includes refining your ethos while training positivity, breath control, visualization, and functional movement. Here is the process:

- When you awake, begin to connect with your breathing and body by performing a quick body scan while breathing deeply. Recite silently to yourself words to this effect: I like myself, I like myself, I've got this, another great day, I am grateful for this day, etc. This immediately grounds you in presence and positivity.

- Your next act when you get out of bed is to get a glass of fresh water, and with gratitude for the water and earth, drink it.

- Now sit in your training space and check in with your ethos: Your ethos (refer back to chapter 3) should be written in a place you can refer to daily—mine is on my iPhone. Simply read the purpose statement and scan your principles. Reflect upon your vision and mission. Consider how you will align with your ethos on this day so that you reinforce it and move the dial toward fulfilling it. This is a good opportunity to deepen your commitment to the important things in your life, or reorient your mind away from things that are distracting you, moving you away from your purpose.

- Perform box breathing for 5 to 20 minutes. Select a ratio that will balance you (1:1:1:1) or charge you up (1:2:2:1). If you are working on a specific breathing pattern, you can do that here instead.

- After the box breathing, it is time to perform your functional movement. This will be one of the pose sequences or spot drill. You can select any other movement practice you would prefer here—like body weight interval or combat conditioning sequences, a jog, or a walk. The key with this part of the ritual is to move the blood and energy in your body. Also it will stimulate and strengthen your spine and nervous system. You will start the day with an integrated body, mind, and spirit.

- After the movement component, sit back down and perform a short visualization session. My preferred method is to visualize my ideal future having accomplished my major life purpose and vision, and then to "dirt dive" my day. In the dirt dive I see myself accomplishing every project, task, and interaction with effortless perfection. You should endeavor to see yourself accomplishing all tasks and projects beyond expectations. All interactions leave you and others elevated. You are positive and in a flow state throughout the day. You have won in your mind.

- You are now ready for your coffee or tea and healthy breakfast. The ritual will help you maintain positive energy and focus as you start your workday.

The Evening Ritual

Whereas the morning ritual is designed to charge you up and ground you for optimal performance in the day, the evening ritual is meant to integrate the positive results of the day, distill the lessons learned, and wind your mind and nervous system down for a great night of sleep. Here is the process:

- Prepare your time and space for the ritual—that means take care of the day's business, put the kids to bed (if applicable), and ensure an uninterrupted time to practice. Have your journal handy.

- Get comfortable and perform 5 to 10 minutes of box breathing. Choose a calming ratio such as 1:0:2:0 or 1:1:2:1.

- Perform a calming sequence such as Peaceful Warrior, Recovering Warrior or Hip Mobility Drill, or if you want just go into Happy Baby or Pidgeon Pose for 5 minutes with a deep awareness of your breath.

- In your mind perform a "recapitulation visualization" where you will visualize yourself back at the start of your day, just after the morning ritual. Moving forward, review all events of the day and mentally note positive interactions and accomplishments. Jot at least three victories down in your journal. Then note the things that didn't go so well. Ponder the lesson, or silver lining, of each event. Write down what you learned, then mentally "let it go" by forgiving yourself and committing to doing better next time. Bottom line: You never want to go to bed with unfinished business or regrets!

- Perform the evening meditation described below, as time allows.

- Drink a nice, cool glass of water with gratitude for your health, for the day, for life, and for anyone or anything else you can think of.

- Go to bed and sleep like a baby!

Evening Meditation: Begin with 5 rounds of alternate nostril breathing. This breathing drill will balance and align the left and right hemispheres of the brain. When finished with that, come back to deep breathing without controlling the breath and notice the shifts in your mind and body. Now reflect on impermanence and the cycle of change that a day represents. One day, one lifetime is what Grandmaster Tadashi Nakamura would tell me, nodding to the cycle of life and how each day is a precious opportunity to be enlightened and aligned in purpose.

Begin to visualize a bright red ball of energy glowing and radiating health near your pelvic floor. Visually create roots that grow from this ball down into the earth. Allow the roots to grow deeper and deeper into the earth, until you have reached the center of the planet and connect to the core. Allow the earth's energy to be drawn up into your body filling you with strength and vitality. Close your practice with gratitude.

The morning and evening rituals will bookend your day in a way that is so powerful that not only will you notice the difference almost immediately, so will everyone else in your life, who will also benefit. I cannot emphasize enough how these rituals are the crux of

SPOT DRILLS

BREATHING DRILLS

Box Breathing

Warrior Breath

Energy Breath

Alternate Nostril Breathing

MENTAL CHECKUP DRILLS

Feed the Courage Wolf

Energizing Visualization

Victorious Warrior Visualization

Future Me Visualization

MOVEMENT DRILLS

Energizing Drill

Hip Mobility Drill

Calming Drill

Body Blast (choose 1 round of a functional drill, or do 50 to 100 of 1 of the following: squats, push-ups, pull-ups, or burpees)

Bring Down the Heavens

Bouncy Breath

Chopping Wood or Musashi Strikes

building your personal practice. Going to a yoga studio a few times a week is great, but doing the morning and evening ritual will have a far more profound and positive impact on your development, and your life!

Spot Drills

Whereas the morning and evening ritual bookend your day and ensure excellence in your personal practice, the spot drills are another way to supercharge your training on a daily basis. The spot drills are designed to do training "on the spot" based upon the time and space you have, and what you feel you need.

For instance, if you are feeling fatigued in midafternoon, you can step away from your desk and perform the spot drill of 1-2-2-1 Breathing or Sun Salutation. If you need to calm yourself and prepare for an important speech, then 5 minutes of box breathing is a nice spot drill. The spot drill is like a Swiss Army knife, a multitool always handy to be certain your integrated training is covering all Five Mountains as you evolve your personal practice. You could schedule these drills, or set reminders to do them throughout the day, or just do them whenever you intuitively feel the need. Above are some of my favorites.

Retreats

Back in my active-duty Navy SEAL days, we did daily ritualistic training unique to preparing for the specialized missions of a SEAL team. But we all looked forward to the next "away time" where we would immerse ourselves 100 percent into learning away from the daily clutter of our lives. On these immersive training adventures we would retrace the basics of whatever skill we were learning, and then take it to a new level, or learn a new skill altogether. We always came home refreshed and energized, even though the training was often grueling for weeks on end.

We achieve this same "away time" immersion in Kokoro Yoga through what we call a retreat. It is important to retreat from busy daily life to immerse yourself in refining a skill or learning something new. The retreat doesn't have to be for yoga; it can come from any of the 5 mountains. For example, some of retreats that I have enjoyed include martial arts, silent meditation, self-defense, emotional therapy, mindfulness, survival, tracking, intuition, memory, and breathing retreats. You can also retreat to charge ahead after a challenge such as a SEALFIT 20X challenge, or a Spartan Race. In any case, the possibilities with the retreat method, as a tool in the integrated training model, are endless. This method of training is incredibly rejuvenating and rewarding...I encourage you to commit to your next one immediately.

STARTING A PERSONAL PRACTICE

If you are new to yoga, as I know many of you are, it can be daunting to figure out how and where to start. Let's just say that you start at the beginning—the beginning that is right for you. For me it was to attend a 60-day Hot Yoga challenge to jump-start my training. Catherine started by leaping right into a 500-hour teacher training! For you it will be different. The key is to fully commit, make it what I call a "burn-your-boats" behind you commitment, the sort where you commit to your significant other, your kids, your inner-sanctum teammates, that you won't let them down.

Commitment gives you the courage to dive in and explore. I would recommend you start by clarifying your personal ethos and begin the morning ritual. In my book *Unbeatable Mind* and the online training program by that name, I have a series of questions and exercises that help you uncover your ethos. I recommend using that process—because it works. At any rate, you need a place to dig your heels into a stand that strengthens your commitment to mastery and resolve to maintain a personal practice day in and day out.

CRAWL, WALK, RUN

In SEAL tactical training we learned to crawl first with a new skill. We were careful not to try to go from zero to hero and risk injury or mission failure. Honing the basics proved to be the most valuable when we actually entered combat. Being able to perform the basics without thinking was crucial to survival and mission success. This is metaphorically true for your yoga practice. Be patient enough to train the basics for far longer than others.

When the basics are mastered, then you will move on to the crawl phase to layer in new skills and knowledge. This is where you will work in greater sync with your teammates. You can eventually run fast with the skill, employing them with precision. But then we would always come back to train the basics again! The brilliance in this method is that it evolves you step-by-step from a place of unconscious incompetence, to conscious incompetence, to conscious competence, and, finally, to unconscious competence where the skills flow with effortlessness. Of course this type of training requires patience and perseverance, two qualities you will need to develop in your practice. It is important to find deep intrinsic motivation, which is why it needs to be grounded in your personal ethos. Relating your training to your ethos is a great intrinsic motivator (i.e., get 1 percent better every day, master yourself so you can serve others, etc.). When you can do this, your personal practice will take on a new level of meaning. Missing it will interfere with your growth as a human, risk your mission and let your team down. We don't do that!

WHERE TO TRAIN

Kokoro Yoga can occur in many places. The most common will be in your home or at work in a spot you have designated or created for your personal practice. I think the home is best because you get to control access and noise (Unless your spouse or kids don't respect your space very well, which is a different issue!). Creating a special place to train and using it every day is powerful. You can include items for you eyes to focus on, such as a candle or an iconic picture. You will have your mat, chair, or bench ready for action. Over time this place will become special to you and have an energy that helps you focus. Try to avoid changing spots or randomly practicing in a different place every time.

Training at work can be a good option if you are lucky enough to work at a conscious company that has dedicated personal development space. Regardless, if you can get access to an empty room, or a park nearby, you can practice. Of course finding a local yoga studio near you is also an excellent option, especially if you resonate with their community. Ideally you will find a combination of these three to provide you ample opportunity to get your practice in every day.

THE THREE MOMENTS

Every practice session has three distinct moments: the beginning, the middle, and the end. The beginning is the preparation and entering into the practice. This will be different for each location. At home the beginning moment will be designed to protect your time and to set up the space. Make sure the phone is on silent and your family or roommate is aware that it is "practice time." It is not a good idea to eat within 30 minutes before a practice. Ensure the room is warm so you won't be distracted by the cold, but not so warm it puts you to sleep. Make sure you have the right tools so you don't have to stop to retrieve them. You get the picture.

The middle moment is the actual practice itself. This is the moment you have been waiting for—so make the most of it—and really practice. A session with a distracted mind, interruptions, chatting with someone, or being crawled on by the kids is not ideal. However don't beat yourself up if you are taken off track by your monkey mind or monkey kids, but use those opportunities to practice a different aspect of your ethos, such as forgiveness, patience, and playfulness.

The end moment is when you wind down and integrate the practice, leaving it with an expression of gratitude and grace. This is where many shortchange themselves. They perform an amazing yoga practice, then as soon as the last pose is done they get up, grab their mat, and check their e-mail. Please don't do that! Take time in the Resting Pose to integrate all that occurred in your practice. The ancient yogis felt that this moment was the most important part of the practice because it allows the benefits to literally sink in at all levels—physical, energetic, mental, wisdom, and bliss—the five dimensional bodies come together as one.

The end moment is also the perfect time to perform visualization work. Generally speaking, we want to start practice with the "hard" work of movement, and then move toward the softer, inner work. Movement precedes breath control, followed by visualization and meditation, in that order. But you may note that I put box breathing before the movement in the sequences. The reason is that I have found it useful to settle and sync the body, mind, and emotions before the movement because it deepens our practice. We are so agitated from the myriad of stressors coming at us day in and out that we can't get enough box breathing in to soothe our nerves and calm our body and our mind. So we kick off our practice with box breathing to ensure that the movement, and entire practice, is stronger.

When you are completely finished, you are still not done. The transition back to the "real" world is also part of your practice. Avoid getting spun up into a conversation right away or checking your e-mail or engaging in some mental drama after your practice. Use the transition time to refine your awareness and grace. Keep quiet, smile, and walk slowly, with awareness. Don't be weird about it, just enjoy the heightened sense of connection and integration, and notice how good it feels. If you do get spun up into another story, notice the difference! Keep in mind that the objective is to develop mental, emotional, and spiritual depth for your personal mastery . . . so that you may fulfill your purpose, live with passion, remain in alignment with your principles, and be of service to others. It makes sense to continue the deep awareness that the practice brought you for as long as possible, doesn't it? Why not make your entire day a practice session? Why not make every action (even every breath) a practice and leave the world better off for it? Why not indeed!

STAYING THE COURSE

Though getting started is a challenge for many, staying the course is often the bigger challenge. We expect immediate results without much effort these days. The good news is that you will see immediate results if by "immediate" you mean 1 to 3 months. Trust me, Kokoro Yoga requires effort, and you will also see results quickly. But after the excitement of the initial positive changes—such as a sense of calm, more control, and more energy—goes away, don't be surprised to find that deeper change seems to evade you. The reason for this is that deeper levels of growth lay dormant until the necessary integration moment occurs— that magical crossroad when the right lessons are learned, and the training penetrates to the right depth, to provide the key that unlocks the new insights or next stage of consciousness.

Positive growth is then suddenly experienced as an "aha" moment, or a sense of knowingness you did not have prior. It just shows up at the right time, often when we are challenged and dig deep. Sometimes we experience it through others by the new way they treat us—with a level of respect we previously didn't experience. They say we have a "look in the eye" that wasn't there before, but of course you can't see it yourself, but you feel it. These are moments to savor and humbly acknowledge that the training is performing its magic. If you are deeply religious, give credit where it is really due, to your Creator.

Bottom line: Transformation is a holistic and nonlinear process that occurs when things line up, when the timing is right.

Another important point I would like to bring up is that we must "translate" our past negative energy into neutral or positive energy in order to transcend to higher stages of consciousness. This means we must overcome shadow self-regrets, shame, and guilt to gain understanding and acceptance of our negative, shadow selves. We do this so that we can end the negative contraction and "graduate" to transcend to higher stages of development. If we try hard to transcend without doing the translation work, we will get pulled back down into negative territory sooner or later. Progress is thwarted by our shadow self, leaving us feeling frustrated and stuck. Translation (shadow work), the gift of Western psychotherapy, and transformation (enlightenment work), the gift of warrior and spiritual practices, conspire together to facilitate our growth to maximum potential as a human. If you just focus on the transcendent practices of meditation, without diving into your shadow self to translate, then transmute mental and emotional negativity, then you will set yourself up for disappointment.

DISCIPLINE, COMPETENCE, CONFIDENCE

Commitment to a daily practice unlocks courage. Courage expresses itself in yoga not as a roar of "I CAN!" but the quiet discipline of just showing up and putting out with a heartfelt effort, every day. Over time that act of discipline leads to a competence in the skills, knowledge, and nuances of the training. Ultimately we gain a concrete confidence in ourselves, a confidence that favorably impacts all that we do. We become more successful, and that success reinforces the confidence. We have unlocked the upward spiral of growth, which has no upper limit.

WHO IS ON YOUR TEAM?

In spite of what you may believe from the movies, a Navy SEAL, or other elite military operator, seeks to master the skills of the warrior not so that they can be a lone operator, but so they can be an effective teammate. Great teams are great because they are filled with individuals working toward greatness. They are willing to align personal needs and desires to the team's mission.

Similarly, in your training, it will help you to find a swim buddy or team to train with. The team-training effect is a critical aspect of the lifestyle I am espousing here. A great team will hold you to a higher standard, call you out on your bull, and offer opportunities to face your fears and develop emotional power. On the contrary, you may find yourself unsupported in your efforts by your supposed team. If that is the case, then I propose you find new teammates. No question, this is an awkward situation if those individuals live under the same roof. Let your newfound confidence and awareness guide the development of a supportive team.

AVOIDING RUTS AND INJURIES

Kokoro Yoga is designed to maximize longevity and to avoid injuries or burnout. The customizable nature of the training and adaptation of the poses and integrated nature will help you maintain a balance throughout your training ups and downs. Having said that, it is possible, if not likely, that eventually injuries may occur. These come from accidents or from dysfunctional movement patterns that grease the groove of an injury. These dysfunctional movement patterns are subtle and hidden from view from us, but can be "outed" by a skilled teacher.

This points to the need to have a teacher to check our work. Attending a yoga studio once a week (or even once a month) to have alignment adjustments and a watchful eye is a good idea. As mentioned above, periodically attending a yoga seminar or retreat is another good idea. Moving into a pose with several repetitions to align your structure, before holding your position, is a tip that Gary Kraftsow taught me. This method will help ferret out dysfunctional movement patterns.

In spite of all the above, what do you do if an injury occurs? First, it helps to assess the magnitude. Maybe it is the Navy SEAL in me, but I have generally noted that many people overestimate the extent of an injury and take unnecessary precautions, sidelining themselves for weeks or months. It is hard to reengage with your personal practice after 3 months on the bench. My Ashtanga teacher, Tim Miller, says that you need to learn the difference between "integrating pain" and "disintegrating pain." Having said that, this is not a recommendation to do anything stupid. Please get injuries examined and follow the advice of your doctor, after checking your intuition and agreeing with it. Remember, the medical docs will always err way on the side of caution to ensure liability coverage. Most of the time you are able to continue training with modifications. An additional professional to consult might be the most experienced yoga professional, chiropractor, or naturopathic doctor in your hood. Don't let injury take you away from your practice—it is part of staying in the game over the long haul.

What if you experience burnout? Burnout is dangerous because it can lead to injury and quitting altogether. Ideally, you will organize your practice with enough variety and regenerative sessions so that you don't experience burnout. But if you do, then what?

Retreat, retreat! Yes, take time to retreat to recharge your batteries. When you begin to feel burnout, instead of taking time off altogether, consider changing things up in your training schedule, and plan an extended period of integrative practice. This can be a day alone, a weekend seminar, or a multiday training. There are an enormous number of excellent seminars and retreats to choose from. Recently I did a 6-day silent Yin Yoga retreat in Hawaii. It completely fired me up to deepen my practice and got me out of a minor rut from the holidays. Finally, to hammer this point home, it helps to check in with your ethos every day to remind yourself why you practice. Maintaining that connection with your "Why" is deeply motivating, providing you the drive and determination to stay the course.

TRUTH, WISDOM, LOVE

So where are we going with all this? What is the destination? There is none. The way of yoga is a journey, not some elusive destination. When we unlock growth, we set ourselves on a path toward an ever-expanding sense of self. The uncanny nature of the growth is that the higher we go up the Five Mountains, the more we can see. The more we see, the more we understand just how little we truly know about the world. Great humility settles in, and we find more grace and joy in the small things in life. Details we didn't even notice as youths, or scoffed at as important business executives, suddenly seem important. And they are.

My directive to you is to you stay focused on the path and not the destination. Put your attention and intention into the daily sharpening of the sword. This is where the good stuff is. You will get glimpses of new plateaus and gain enlightening insights to guide future steps. Day by day, step-by-step, that divine heart of your inner warrior, your spirit, and the witness to your life, will begin to merge with your physical heart. You will be consumed with the courage wolf and positivity will be your constant companion as you experience ever-expanding waves of truth, wisdom, and love. Your thoughts and actions will be filled with passion, directed toward purpose, guided by worthy principles, and backed by your stand. You will move as fast as the wind, be as quiet as the forest, as daring as fire, and as immovable as a mountain itself.

Life will become about finding perfection in the moment, about discovering truth, unlocking the capacity to love, and to live with wisdom in deep connection to all of life. This is our journey, our way. It is time that we all step into our uniqueness, gain mastery over our body and minds, and allow our spirits to speak to the world. It is time to fulfill our purpose with passion, and live with honor, courage, and commitment.

We are deeply humbled that you have chosen to join this journey.

FUNCTIONAL CONDITIONING

The following functional conditioning movements are for the Fit Warrior sequences. You will choose a handful of these to add to your practice. Appendix B has combat conditioning movements, and Appendix C has some combinations of both fitness and combat conditioning movements to get you started. Change it up and have fun with these!

For more guidance on proper technique and methodology for functional fitness, see www.sealfit.com/videos and my book *8 Weeks to SEALFIT*.

Remember the golden rule of virtuosity when it comes to maximizing your conditioning modules: good form is the first priority and intensity comes second. In other words, don't make the mistake of compromising good technique to bang out a few more reps.

PUSH-UPS

Standard Push-up

- Elbows close to body, core engaged.
- Chest touches ground, elbows locked out at top.

Scaled Push-up

- Hand position elevated on a box or wall.
- Chest touches box or wall.

Plyometric Push-up

- Explosive UP, hands and feet leave the ground.
- In place or moving across the floor forward or backward.

Dive Bomber Push-ups

- Top of push-up, send hips up, moving in a V.
- Scoop the chest down and forward low, with hips following. Lock arms, then reverse to the start.

Clapping Push-ups

- Explosive UP, hands leave the ground, and clap in front of or behind the body.

Alligator Push-ups

- Offset grip (fore and aft), do a push-up, crawl forward, and repeat on the other side.

Hand-Placement Variations

- Diamond (formed with thumbs and index fingers touching).
- Wide.
- On fists.
- Offset (fore and aft).

Wave-offs (Arm Haulers)

- On belly, arms, and legs lifted. Hands touch in front, sweep back, and touch behind back.

Static Plank Hold

- Either top of push-up position or on elbows with straight body or in pike as lean and rest.

Single Arm

- Center-weighted arm under body, other behind back.
- Can scale on a box or well-secured chair.

Handstand Push-up

- Upside down against wall, arms locked out.
- Lower with control to touch head to ground or elevated pad. Lift back up to straight arms.
- Can scale with feet on a box and the body in pike position.
- Handstand hold is also an option.

SQUATS AND JUMPS

Standard Squat

- Feet shoulder width, initiate by driving hips back. Weight on heels.
- Proud chest, eyes forward, knees out, tracking over toes.
- Bottom is reached when the hip crease is below the top of the knee.

Jump Squat

- Accelerate through the top, hips open, feet leave the ground.
- Soft landing, core engaged.

Squat Hold

- Hold at the bottom to work mobility or slightly above parallel to work strength.

Single Leg Squat (Pistol)

- Drive hips back, unweighted leg in front.
- Send weight back.

Tuck Jumps

- Jump straight up, pulling knees up high.
- Quiet, springy landing.

Star Jump

- Squat down, touch hands to floor.
- Spring up with the feet leaving the floor and arms out, body forms an X.

Jumping Jacks

- Stand up straight, with arms at the side.
- Jump feet and arms wide, with elbows bending at the top.

Froggies

- Squat and touch fingertips to the ground.
- Jump into the top of a wide-stance jumping jack.

LUNGES

Standard Lunge

- Big step forward, knee tracks over foot.
- Back leg lightly touches the ground.
- Eyes forward, upright torso.
- Return to standing.

Jump Lunges

- Jump from one lunge to another with core engagement and control.

Walking Lunges

- Connect lunges to move forward or backward.

CORE

Sit-ups

- On back, soles of feet together.
- Engage core and lift to sitting.

Flutter Kicks

- On back, fists under glutes, legs straight.
- Lift and lower legs, keeping them straight (scissor).

Plank Toe Taps

- On elbows, body straight.
- Lift one leg and tap toes to heel
- Lower and repeat with the other.

Side Hip Raises

- On one elbow or locked out arm, body straight, side torso facing down.
- Lower hip to tap the ground and raise to return to a straight body.

Bicycle Crunches

- Sit in a V, touch right elbow to left knee while extending left leg.
- Repeat.

Leg Levers and Holds

- On back, fists under glutes, legs straight.
- Lift and lower straight legs or hold at various heights.

Supermans

- On belly, arms outreached, palms face each other or down.
- Lift arms and legs together, engaging core and reaching legs back.

Jump Throughs

- Pike Position/Downward-Facing Dog.
- Bend knees, lift heels, look forward.
- Jump feet through to sitting, crossing the ankles when the feet are passing between the arms.

MULTIJOINT MOVEMENTS

Down-Ups

- Drop to your back or belly (spontaneous choice).
- Jump back up to a choice combat stance.
- Repeat ad infinitum.

Burpees

1. Hands to ground.
2. Feet jump out to top of push-up position.
3. Chest to ground.
4. Lift chest, jump feet to the bottom of a squat.
5. Jump up, open hips, claps hands over head.

8-Count Body Builders

1. Hands to ground.
2. Feet jump out to top of push-up position.
3. Chest to ground.
4. Top of push-up.
5. Jump feet wide.
6. Jump feet back to normal push-up position.
7. Jump feet to the bottom of a squat.
8. Jump up, open hips, claps hands over head.

Mountain Climbers

- Top of push-up position.
- Right foot jumps to outside of right hand.
- Left foot jumps to outside of left hand as right foot jumps back to starting position.
- Repeat.

COMBAT CONDITIONING

We talked about "combat conditioning" in chapter 4: It's a fantastic way to insert a fun and highly charged aerobic element using offensive and protective movements into your Kokoro Yoga routine. I'll say this again because it's so important: You don't need to have a martial arts background to throw a few punches and kicks. Throwing some punches and kicks (the essence of combat conditioning) can be done as a stand-alone workout or inserted as a conditioning module in your routine.

The combat conditioning module is not a requirement, of course. Rather, it's offered as a method to include a specific brand of heart-pounding cardio into the 1 hour (or 30 minutes) of time that you have to train on a jam-packed day. Combat conditioning moves can also be intermixed with functional fitness moves. As long as you're consistent in changing things up, you'll avoid the rut of stagnation that can occur from doing the exact same routine every time you train. Constantly varying your functional conditioning is a way to shock the body into delivering the highest return on your investment when it comes to physiological response to your training.

Kicks

■ Front: lift knee, kick quickly straight ahead through the ball of the foot (vary the height), quick recoil.

■ Side: lift knee, kick to side through the heel (quick out-in).

Punches

■ Straight punch: fists, arms up to protect head, offset stance, drive rear side arm forward, rotate hips.

■ Jab: fists, arms up to protect head, offset stance, drive front side arm forward.

■ Hook: bent elbow punch from the side, use hips and upper-back muscles.

Ducks and Feints

■ Side-to-side moves, squat, head moves.

Sprawl

■ Jump the legs back.

■ Arch the back, hands to ground, control the descent with the chest striking first and contact rolling down the front of the body (like the rockers on a rocking horse).

CONDITIONING MODULES

Picking and choosing from the movements listed in Appendix A and Appendix B, you can craft your own conditioning modules that you can insert into the middle of a Kokoro Yoga session. The following workout patterns can be used as templates.

10! UP or DOWN

- Pick 2 or more movements.
- 10 reps each, then 9 each . . . continuing down to 1 each.
- Can start at 1 and work up the ladder as well.
- Can do 10 of 1 movement and 1 of another and work the ladders in opposite directions.

x Rounds of y Reps

- 5 rounds of 20 reps each.
- 3 rounds of 15 reps each.

AMRAP

- As many rounds as possible (in X time).
- For example, 12 minutes AMRAP of 5 burpees + 5 Mountain Climbers.

EMOM

- Every minute on the minute.

Roll the Dice

- Pick 2 to 6 movements and assign dice numbers.
- Roll the dice and choose the corresponding movement.
- Roll it again for rep count, double or triple it.

A Few Sample Modules:

10! UP: standard push-ups, L+R straight punches, sit-ups

5 rounds of 20 reps each of: jumping jacks, squats, Supermans, lunges

AMRAP 8 minutes: 4 burpees, 6 front kicks, 8 wave-offs, 10 Mountain Climbers

EMOM 10 minutes: 3 star jumps, 4 dive bomber push-ups, 5 2-count flutter kicks (scale up with 4-count flutter kicks)

MARK DIVINE

A *New York Times, Wall Street Journal,* and Amazon.com bestselling author, Mark Divine is the founder of SEALFIT and Unbeatable Mind. Mark served for twenty years as a Navy SEAL, retiring as a Commander in 2011. He is an accomplished martial artist with black belts in Seido and Goju Ryu Karate, as well as military hand-to-hand combat certification in SCARS/San Soo Kng Foo and a senior ranking in Saito Ninjutsu.

Mark came to yoga from the martial arts in 1999, studying with Ashtanga Yoga's Tim Miller, where he received teacher training in the first and second series. He later received a 500-hour teaching certification from Gary Kraftkow's American ViniYoga Academy. In 2007 Mark created the innovative Kokoro Yoga program to train Navy SEAL and other SOF candidates the science of mental development through SEALFIT. Since then, he has trained thousands from all walks of life to embrace the full spectrum of physical, mental, emotional, and spiritual training that yoga offers.

CATHERINE DIVINE

After years of the stress of work as a professional cook, Catherine found in yoga a path toward healing. Yoga soon became her medicine as well as the focus of a new path in life. She is now an experienced teacher and spiritual activist, flowing with enthusiasm for the healing properties yoga brings to each individual. In collaboration with stepfather Mark Divine, the founder of Kokoro Yoga, Catherine is the head facilitator for programming, teacher training, and yoga retreats for the program. Catherine has multiple teaching certifications and has trained in various styles under some of the best teachers in the world, including Tim Miller and Gary Kraftsow. Her key focus as a teacher is to bring a community together under the common thread of the Peaceful Warrior, seeking compassion, love, and environmental awareness.

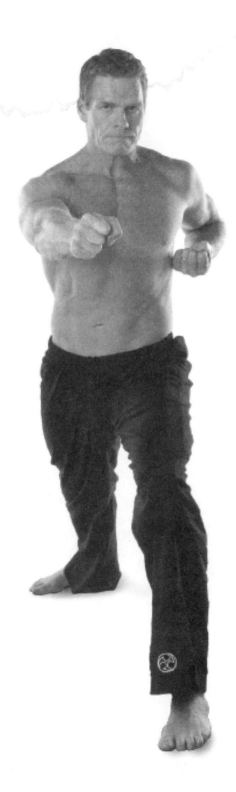

We Hope You Enjoyed

KOKORO
YOGA

You're well on your way to a strong flexible body and unbeatable mind.

To help you experience even more benefits from your Kokoro Yoga practice—including stronger core, leaner physique, reduced stress, enhanced focus, and much more, **we're gifting you a free trial membership to Kokoro Yoga Online.**

Enhance your practice by participating in live streaming events and watching supplemental videos from your tablet or phone plus exciting special offers.

VISIT WWW.WARRIORYOGA.COM and sign up using this special coupon code.

KOYOGAFREE